Letters *from* Pharmacy Residents

Navigating Your Career

EDITORS

SARA J. WHITE, RPh, MS, FASHP
Director of Pharmacy (Ret.)
Stanford Hospital and Clinics
Past President, ASHP
Palo Alto, California
Faculty, ASHP Foundation's Pharmacy Leadership
    Academy

HAROLD N. GODWIN, RPh, MS, FASHP, FAPhA
Professor Emeritus
University of Kansas School of Pharmacy
Past President, ASHP, ACPE, APhA
Overland Park, Kansas
Faculty, ASHP Foundation's Pharmacy
Leadership Academy

SUSAN TEIL BOYER, RPh, MS, FASHP
Senior Consultant, ASHP Consulting
Past Board Member, ASHP
Tacoma, Washington

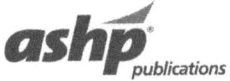

Any correspondence regarding this publication should be sent to the publisher, American Society of Health-System Pharmacists, 4500 East West Highway, Suite 900, Bethesda, MD 20814, attention: Special Publishing.

The information presented herein reflects the opinions of the contributors and advisors. It should not be interpreted as an official policy of ASHP or as an endorsement of any product.

Because of ongoing research and improvements in technology, the information and its applications contained in this text are constantly evolving and are subject to the professional judgment and interpretation of the practitioner due to the uniqueness of a clinical situation. The editors and ASHP have made reasonable efforts to ensure the accuracy and appropriateness of the information presented in this document. However, any user of this information is advised that the editors and ASHP are not responsible for the continued currency of the information, for any errors or omissions, and/or for any consequences arising from the use of the information in the document in any and all practice settings. Any reader of this document is cautioned that ASHP makes no representation, guarantee, or warranty, express or implied, as to the accuracy and appropriateness of the information contained in this document and specifically disclaims any liability to any party for the accuracy and/or completeness of the material or for any damages arising out of the use or non-use of any of the information contained in this document.

Editorial Project Manager: Ruth Bloom
Production Director: Johnna Hershey
Cover & Page Design: David Wade

Library of Congress Cataloging-in-Publication Data

Names: White, Sara J., 1945- editor. | Godwin, Harold N., editor. | Boyer, Susan Teil, editor. | American Society of Health-System Pharmacists, issuing body.
Title: Letters from pharmacy residents : navigating your career/editors, Sara J. White, Harold N. Godwin, Susan Teil Boyer.
Description: Bethesda, MD: ASHP, [2018] | Includes bibliographical references.
Identifiers: LCCN 2018003696 | ISBN 9781585286089 (pbk.)
Subjects: |MESH: Pharmacy Residencies |Pharmacy--methods |Vocational Guidance | Collected Correspondence
Classification: LCC RS110 | NLM WZ 112.5.P4 | DDC 615.1071/55--dc23 LC record available at https://lccn.loc.gov/2018003696

ISBN: 978-1-58528-608-9

Printed in Canada

10 9 8 7 6 5 4 3 2 1

DEDICATION

This book is dedicated to all those pharmacists who so selflessly have been Residency Program Directors and rotation preceptors.

The profession and our patients continue to benefit from the ongoing improvement of pharmacy care and services that residency-trained pharmacists often develop and implement.

ACKNOWLEDGMENTS

We are indebted to the Residency Program Directors and Pharmacy Leaders who recommended these residents who had recently completed their programs to be letter contributors. These young pharmacists were wonderful to work with and readily shared their residency experiences so others could benefit from them.

We want to express our sincere appreciation to Beth Campbell, Ruth Bloom, Johnna Hershey, and their colleagues in ASHP Publishing for their guidance and patience throughout the development and production of this book.

TABLE OF CONTENTS

Letters

FOREWORD

Janet A. Silvester, PharmD, MBA, FASHP and

Paul W. Abramowitz, PharmD, ScD (hon), FASHP

Although residency program accreditation began more than 50 years ago, residency training in the form of internships began in the 1930s. Harvey A. K. Whitney and Edward C. Watts led the first internship program at the University of Michigan in Ann Arbor. Since our founding 75 years ago, ASHP has been faithfully committed to postgraduate residency training. The contributions of residency training to pharmacy practice advancement have been significant, especially in the early years in hospitals, and are considered foundational to strong pharmacy patient care in all healthcare settings today. ASHP staff have led and championed residency accreditation advancements since its inception. These individuals include John Oliver (1962–1965), Warren E. McConnell (1966–1977), Max D. Ray (1977–1985), Donald E. Letendre (1986–2001), Janet L. Teeters (2002–2014), Katrin Fulginiti (2015–2017), and Janet A. Silvester (2013–present).[1]

The ASHP Minimum Standard for Pharmacy Internships in Hospitals was developed and approved in 1951.[2] However, many attempts to create an internship accreditation process fell short. The term *residency* was adopted in 1962 when a group of pharmacy leaders envisioned the first accreditation process and developed the standards that would support accreditation site surveys. The hospitals that provided internships were then encouraged to apply for accreditation. The first official accreditation site survey was conducted on May 21–22, 1963, at Jefferson Medical College Hospital in Philadelphia. By August 1964, there were 32 accredited pharmacy residency programs in 31 hospitals. The original ASHP- accredited residency programs were an Army medical center, four U.S. Public Health Services hospitals, nine Veterans Affairs hospitals, 12 university medical centers, and six community hospitals.[3]

During the early period of residency training, pharmacy practice and, therefore, residency training, focused largely on the preparation and distribution of pharmaceuticals. The essential leadership training and related skills needed for hospital pharmacy practice advancement were also an important focus of the program. During this period, most pharmacists worked in a central pharmacy and communicated with physicians and nurses largely by telephone. Unit dose and intravenous admixture programs were rare.

As the profession moved from the 1960s into the 1970s, emphasis on the patient and management of drug therapy became a feature of a growing number of residency programs. This evolution was reflected in changes in the Accreditation Standard for Pharmacy Residency in a Hospital in 1974.[4] Some residency programs, such as the University of Michigan Hospitals and Clinics, the University of Kentucky Hospital, and the University of Cincinnati Hospitals, concentrated their residency training on the provision of clinical pharmacy services. These early *clinical residencies* were often associated with the postgraduate doctor of pharmacy programs at their respective colleges of pharmacy. This change provided a major stimulus to the clinical pharmacy movement. Other programs such as those at the University of Kansas, the Ohio State University, and the University of Wisconsin combined their residency programs focused on management and leadership with the Master of Science degrees at their respective colleges of pharmacy. These programs produced a large number of future pharmacy directors. In 1980, the first Accreditation Standard for Residency Training in Clinical Pharmacy was released.[5] Therefore, for a time, ASHP had two types of residency programs, hospital pharmacy residencies and clinical pharmacy residencies. The ASHP Commission on Credentialing was created in the late 1970s to administer the entire accreditation process.

As the focus on clinical pharmacy practice continued to grow, services within hospitals also matured. The complexity of medication therapy and the increasing involvement of pharmacists in optimizing care outcomes highlighted the need for pharmacy specialists. This realization resulted in the development of the first Accreditation Standard for Specialized Pharmacy Residency Training[6] and the Supplemental Standard and Learning Objectives for Residency Training in Psychiatric Pharmacy Practice[7] in 1980. This model of specialized residency training quickly grew to include specialty residencies including internal medicine, critical care, drug information, geriatrics, oncology, pediatrics, clinical kinetics, nuclear, nutritional support, and others.

At the 1985 Hilton Head Conference[8] on Directions for Clinical Practice in Pharmacy and the 1989 National Residency Preceptors Conference,[9] recommendations to merge the hospital and clinical residency standards were made; in 1991 the Accreditation Standard for Residency in Pharmacy Practice was approved.[10] The use of the term *pharmacy practice* was purposeful in that there was agreement to no longer distinguish between clinical pharmacy practice and general hospital practice. By 1992, all previous hospital and clinical residencies became residencies in pharmacy practice. The standard for these new residencies in pharmacy practice identified four areas of required training: acute care, ambulatory care, drug information and drug use policy development, and practice management.

To respond to the need for residencies in additional practice settings, goals and objectives were developed for home care, long-term care, and managed care practice settings. The development of these goals and objectives was performed in cooperation with the American Society of Consultant Pharmacists and the Academy of Managed Care Pharmacists. The ASHP Section of Home Care Practitioners (later to become the ASHP Section of Ambulatory Care Practitioners) supported the goals and objectives for home care. A need for the use of instructional design methodology in the development of educational requirements for residency was identified. A grant from the ASHP Research and Education Foundation funded the development of the Residency Learning System (RLS), which outlined a systematic approach to residency training. This system was tested during 1994–1995 and unveiled at the national residency conference in 1996.

In 2005, new accreditation standards resulted in the replacement of pharmacy practice residencies with *postgraduate year one (PGY1)* pharmacy residencies and specialized residencies with *postgraduate year two (PGY2)* pharmacy residencies. The PGY1 residency became a prerequisite for PGY2 residency program admission. Concerns about the readiness of new graduates to care for the increasing complexity of both hospitalized and ambulatory care patients led to residency training as the bridge between formal education and practice. ASHP contracted with the National Matching Service (NMS) in 1994 as the number of residency programs and applicants rose significantly. In 2007, participation in the Matching Service was a requirement for all programs. As the profession of pharmacy evolved further, the ASHP House of Delegates in 2007 approved a policy that stated that by the year 2020, all new pharmacy graduates should be required to complete a PGY1 residency to provide direct patient care.

To meet this goal, ASHP and the profession greatly increased its efforts to expand the number of accredited residency programs and the number of residents per program to meet this demand. The capacity of residency training has since increased by an average of 9% per year for the last five years, with the number of residents in training programs increasing from 2,998 in 2012 to 4,586 today.

To assist in this effort, the ASHP Research and Education Foundation began funding residency expansion grants in 2011. ASHP currently accredits approximately 2,300 residency programs including 30 different PGY2 specialty areas of practice. PGY1 programs now exist in hospitals, clinics, community pharmacy, and managed care practice settings. More than 4,500 residents will graduate in 2018.

Residency training as envisioned by Harvey A.K. Whitney and other leaders is often cited as one of the most important factors in advancing the profession of pharmacy from where it was in the 1960s to today. We believe it will continue to do so.

REFERENCES

1.   Zellmer WA. Creation of the ASHP residency accreditation program: the choices of early leaders. *Am J Health-Syst Pharm*. 2014; 71:1183-1189.

2.   Etheldreda M Sr. Report of committee on minimum standards. *Bull Am Soc Hosp Pharm*. 1951; 8:319–21.

3.   Clark T. Celebrating 50 years of advancement in pharmacy residency training. *Am J Health-Syst Pharm*. 2014; 71(14):1190-1195.

4.   Accreditation Standard for Pharmacy residency in a Hospital. *Am J Health-Syst Pharm*. 1975; 32:192-198.

5.   ASHP Accreditation Standard for Residency Training in Clinical Pharmacy. *Am J Health-Syst Pharm*. 1980; 37:1223-1228.

6.   ASHP Accreditation Standard for Specialized Pharmacy Residency Training. *Am J Health-Syst Pharm*. 1980; 37:1229-1232.

7.   ASHP Supplementary Standard and Learning Objectives for Residency Training in Psychiatric Pharmacy Practice. *Am J Health-Syst Pharm*. 1980; 37:1232-1234.

8.   Directions for Clinical Practice in Pharmacy. Proceedings of an invitational conference conducted by the ASHP Research and Education Foundation and the American Society of Hospital Pharmacists. *Am J Health-Syst Pharm*. 1985; 42:1287-1342.

9.   Directions for Postgraduate Pharmacy Residency Training. Proceedings of the 1989 National Residency Preceptors Conference conducted by the American Society of Hospital Pharmacists. *Am J Health-Syst Pharm*. 1990; 47:85-126.

10. ASHP Accreditation Standard for Residency in Pharmacy Practice. *Am J Health-Syst Pharm*. 1992; 49: 146-153.

PREFACE

For this publication, we contacted a representative and varied group of Residency Program Directors, Directors of Pharmacy, and Chief Pharmacy Officers from across the country. We asked for a recommendation and introduction to one of their recent past residents to be a possible letter writer. Thus, *Letters from Pharmacy Residents: Navigating Your Career* contains 33 contributions—sharing personal experiences in seeking a residency, completing a residency, finding a first pharmacist position, and starting a career journey.

We believe the best thing we ever did was to complete a residency. We developed the confidence, knowledge, skills, and abilities to do whatever we liked throughout our careers and lives. Even decades after finishing our programs, in sticky situations we often ask ourselves, "What would Clif do?" Clifton J. Latiolais was the Director of Pharmacy and a mentor to all of us during and after our residencies at Ohio State. As a resident you become part of a network of program participants that provides you with contacts, mentors, information, and assistance as your career progresses. Residency programs have a legacy that benefits you for the rest of your career.

Over the past four decades we have been Big L (formal) leaders in community and major health systems as well as local, state, and national professional organization presidents (ASHP, ACPE [Accreditation Council for Pharmacy Education] and APhA [American Pharmacists Association]). We have also served on and chaired state boards of pharmacy. Moreover, we have conducted residencies throughout our careers because we are committed to training future pharmacists not only as **Big L** leaders but as **little l** leaders on their shift or in their practice to continue the evolution of pharmacy services on behalf of patients. We are attempting to *pay forward to others* so they, too, have successful and rewarding careers.

The pharmacy service evolution during our careers has evolved dramatically to include intravenous admixture programs, pharmacy technicians, unit dose systems, clinical pharmacy, ambulatory patient profiles and counseling, computerization, automation, computerized physician order entry, electronic medical records, and managing a variety of medication-intensive disease states. The future services that pharmacists will perform will be determined by residency-trained pharmacists.

Deciding whether to do a residency and getting an interview and then successfully matching is very challenging in today's competitive environment but very doable with planning and persistence. The application process alone involves decisions such as the size of program; double-digit residents or two to three; type of residency site; community practice or health system; location; urban or rural site; academic or not; availability of postgraduate year 2 (PGY2) specialty programs; and who to ask for references. Making the most of the Residency Showcase at the ASHP's Midyear Clinical Meeting is a good investment. (If possible, consider attending the meeting the year prior to applying.) Asking for assistance in preparing and practicing for interviews is wise. Once you are successful in matching, you should then think about which elective rotations you might want and how to maximize the program. It is recommended that you get outside your comfort zone for maximum learning. In residency programs, you will get experience working with different people as preceptors, so perfecting your communication skills will benefit you in your career and life. About half way through your residency, you will need to decide whether to go on to a PGY2 or find your first full-time position. Regardless of your choice, you should think about how to maximize your career and integrate your personal life with your career.

In addition to the various aspects of residencies just described, you will find letters that specifically relate decisions and experiences about the following:

- deciding to do a residency versus a PhD
- deciding not to do a PGY2
- being married and doing a residency
- having a baby during a residency
- maximizing unique learning opportunities such as a nursing strike
- coping with the complete pharmacy departmental leadership team turnover
- being the chief resident
- coping with obstacles and disappointments
- encountering and dealing with healthcare issues affecting you or a loved one during your program

Letters from Pharmacy Residents: Navigating Your Career joins Susan A. Cantrell, Sara J. White, and Bruce E. Scott's *Letters to a Young Pharmacist: Sage Advice on Life and Career from Extraordinary Pharmacists* (mid-career to veterans) and Susan A. Cantrell and Sara J. White's *Letters from Rising Pharmacy Stars: Advice on Creating and Advancing Your Career in a Changing Profession* (pharmacists with at least 10 years of practice). Both ASHP-published books were the brainchild of Susan A. Cantrell who had read books written by Ellyn Spragins, which featured authors writing letters to their younger selves. Susan talked to Sara about using the concept for pharmacists, which resulted in the first two *Letters* books. Because Susan was busy with a new position, she declined to be a co-editor for this publication so Harold N. Godwin and Susan Teil Boyer were recruited as they have conducted residencies throughout their careers and have been active in promoting the pharmacy profession in various leadership roles.

We rarely find anyone who has regrets once they have finished a residency; residencies are programs that keep giving throughout one's career and life.

We hope you find these letters helpful on your journey.

Sara J. White, Harold N. Godwin, and Susan Teil Boyer

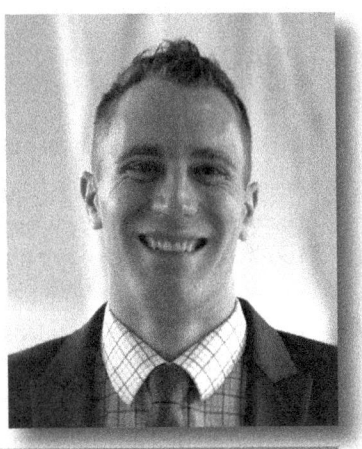

Andrew Albanese
PharmD, MBA

It Is All about Practice and Attitude

As a resident, Andrew had a strong curiosity about learning new things. He is professional and thoughtful in his approach and is always open to feedback. Andrew is dedicated to the profession, and it shows through his involvement with national and local pharmacy organizations. His transition from administrative resident to Ambulatory Pharmacy Operations Manager was seamless because Andrew was ready for the challenge. Andrew is energetic and has a thirst to learn more and grow both professionally and personally.

Andrew is the Ambulatory Pharmacy Operations Manager at Oregon Health and Sciences University Health System, Portland. Andrew completed his postgraduate year 1 (PGY1)/PGY2 accredited health-system pharmacy administration residency at the Oregon Health and Sciences University Health System and his PGY1 accredited pharmacy residency at Peace Health Southwest Washington Medical Center, Vancouver. He received his BS degree in Pre-Pharmacy at Oregon State University, Corvallis and his PharmD degree at Oregon Health and Sciences University and Oregon State University College of Pharmacy, Portland. He earned his MBA from Oregon State University.

Andrew's advice is: **Residency has been designed to make you better—to break down bad habits, to identify strengths as well as weaknesses, and to better know yourself and what you need to succeed.**

Dear Pharmacy Colleague,

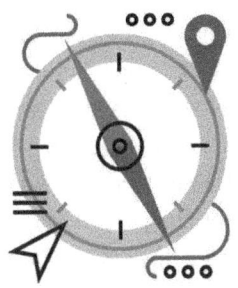

I am one of the few lucky ones who completed three years of pharmacy residency. And no, I did not have to redo any years or get dismissed from a program. I chose this fate! Many, and especially those who have completed a residency, have asked me why. Many people have also asked if I'm right in the head, and my response to them is: practice and attitude.

PRACTICE

Malcolm Gladwell, in his popular book *Outliers,* describes that 10,000 hours of practice is the essence of mastery and success. One doesn't just wake up and perform brain surgery, but must practice and hone the skill for 10,000 hours before mastery. This theory isn't perfect; genetics help in most cases, but this theory applies to pharmacy too. To equate this to our pharmacy world, a third-year pharmacy student doesn't walk out of a clinical therapeutics lecture and practice as a pharmacist on an intensive care unit (ICU). He or she needs thousands of hours in clinical- and ICU-specific experiences to become a master and manage medications that keep people who are close to death from dying. As a student looking at a pharmacy practice residency, and then as a resident looking at an administration residency, I knew I needed to be honed and humbled so I could rise to new heights of mastery!

"Practice isn't the thing you do once you're good. It's the thing you do that makes you good." —Malcolm Gladwell

Let's crunch the numbers. Two years of residency, working—let's be realistic—at least 60 hours a week is 6,240 hours. You are two-thirds of the way there! I just added another 3,120 hours for good measure and graduated ready for anything (which, unfortunately, was not the case). That is the point of residency, and how residency should be framed. Residency programs give you many opportunities to practice as a pharmacist to aid and accelerate the process to mastery.

So, my first message to you is grab your career by the horns and pursue a residency. Who doesn't want to be a master ... sooner!

My journey was quite practice heavy between my PGY1 at Peace Health Southwest in Vancouver, Washington, and then a two-year health-system pharmacy administration residency with a concurrent MBA program at Oregon Health and Science University. It was a long journey with more practice opportunities than I can count. I look back on those trials, challenges, successes, and failures fondly. The opportunity to practice is what got me to where I am today.

Practice does more than hone your skills. How do you know you are good at something? How do you know what you are not naturally gifted in? Residency is a fire-breathing mirror that shows a reflection of things you are naturally good at and areas that you are not. Without practice, without opportunities to learn, you will not find the answers to these important interpersonal questions. During my first year of clinical pharmacy practice residency, my co-residents and I were presented with options for residency projects that included new clinical services in ambulatory clinics or collaborative practice agreements—the cool pharmacy stuff. However, at the end of the project presentations, my residency program director told us that someone would have to choose the management operations project to implement USP <797> standards in the not-so-new intravenous (IV) room. Although I had dreams of being the coolest emergency department pharmacist in the Pacific Northwest, I knew that USP <797> standards really needed to be implemented. Previously I had enjoyed working on projects that impacted many people, so I decided to step up and volunteered to implement USP <797> for my project. Midway through the project (when I was presenting and asking my director for funds), I realized I really liked working with technicians and pharmacists to implement these standards. I enjoyed assimilating and presenting data to request resources. Those things sound boring to most people, but they were like working through a puzzle to me. In addition to this project, I presented a re-validation and expansion to the technician-checking-technician program to the Washington State Department of Health, Washington Board of Pharmacy. It was exhilarating! They liked it, it was successful, and I was extremely happy about how I was impacting patients. That night I looked in the mirror and realized I was much better at presentations, data crunching, and leading people than being a cool emergency department pharmacist. And oddly enough, I was OK with it.

Without practice, without being thrown into the fire, without sweating in front of a board asking for their approval, I would have never unearthed my talents this early in my career. Residency provides this experience. *Residency shows you where you are naturally gifted.*

On the flipside, residency shows you where you are not naturally gifted. It shows you your weaknesses and, if blessed with good mentors, helps you mitigate them. We are all human, and we all have weaknesses or areas that we really don't want to spend time in. The worst thing you could do is claim they do not exist by ignoring them.

Early in my health-system pharmacy administration residency, I realized I struggled with going too fast with projects and not uncovering the important details. For example, my preceptor had me facilitate a Kaizen event to optimize our operating room (OR) pharmacy workflows. I would present ideas that I felt were very good and go over my plan with him, and then he would poke holes and identify details I hadn't known existed or considered. Drilling down all of the many components did not come naturally to me. So what did I do? I strategized to mitigate this weakness. I quickly picked up that he would ask the question "Why?" countless times to unearth every detail. I took notes on how he approached projects; I emulated him at every possible opportunity. I learned and practiced things that came naturally to my preceptor. Will I ever be as good as he is at identifying every possible detail about a project or workflow? Simply . . . the answer is no. And it's OK as long as I learn how he uses his natural ability and mimic his techniques that work well with my strengths.

During my second year of administration residency, my main project was to create a business plan for a home infusion pharmacy and receive approval from hospital administration. The skills I learned about strengthening my not-so-natural gifts served me well. I knew that, alone, I wouldn't even come close to identifying crucial details for the project's success. From my previous learning opportunities, it was clear I needed experts who knew all of the details. Fortunately, meeting with people, presenting, and getting others excited about a project is one of my gifts so getting buy-in was a fun experience; coupled with knowledge of key details, this ultimately led to success. If I hadn't completed my inpatient operations residency, I would not have known where I could or could not perform using my own natural ability. For the final business plan and presentation to the C-suite, my director poured over the details to ensure that I, a mere pharmacy resident, would be ready for my biggest and most important presentation in my young career. This practice was essential to the project's success. Because she invested in me and helped me identify my strengths and weaknesses, the proposal was a success. *A good life lesson is to always surround yourself with people who are better than you, especially at those things you are not gifted in.*

Whenever you practice, introspection is critical. What would I do differently if I got to do it all over again? I would have invested more in my relationships with my co-residents. Being the administration resident comes with a lot of "extra opportunities." I said yes to many of them and gave up times when I could have been building relationships with my fellow residents. Never minimize the importance and value of relationships.

ATTITUDE

The second message is that your attitude affects more than you know. I had many mentors say my positive attitude was borderline annoying, which I understand, but what it does for me far outweighs what other people may think. Life is going to come at you and try to take you down regardless of your attitude, so why not enjoy the journey?

A genuinely positive attitude is rather rare in today's society. Many see it as being naïve or weak, which discourages people from nurturing this valuable characteristic. Don't listen to the haters! During a PGY1 evaluation, my preceptor told me that I needed to stop being so positive. Being positive was considered annoying in the medical world versus a more "non-positive" attitude—the meaning of which still eludes me. I agree with my preceptor that being genuine is important. But having energy and using it to produce a lot of work and get through challenging times is not something that anyone should *stop* doing.

What did a positive attitude do for me during residency? During the long hours and late nights of residency I would remind myself, despite this feeling of physical and mental exhaustion, that I had one of the most unique jobs in the world. My job is to learn and accept feedback and words of wisdom from people who are smarter and more experienced as well as amazing leaders. How could I *not* have a positive attitude?

I get to do what I love every day and get better at it. When I framed my residency experience this way in my mind, the challenges and long hours didn't seem quite so bad.

Remember, *practice and attitude.* Residency has been designed to make you better. To break down bad habits, to identify strengths as well as weaknesses, and to better know yourself and what you need to succeed. If what I have described seems like an adventure you would like to embark on, please complete a residency! And why not have a great attitude? Residency is like a running a marathon. You are sore and tired, and often question why you are doing this to yourself. But, like running a marathon—once completed—you look back at the experience as life changing.

Good luck on your adventures!

Andrew

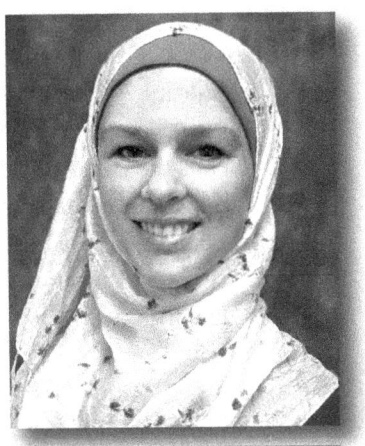

Kallie A. Amer
PharmD

Finding a New Equilibrium as a Resident with a New Son

Kallie is a thoughtful, reflective professional who impresses people with her insight into values and beliefs that drive her decision making. Her letter presents a meaningful perspective for individuals early in their career path who are married, who are parents, and who are also faced with not being matched.

Kallie is currently a Transitions of Care Pharmacist at Cedars-Sinai Medical Center, Los Angeles, California. She completed an accredited postgraduate year 1 (PGY1) pharmacy practice residency at St. John Hospital and Medical Center, Detroit, Michigan and a PGY2 transitions of care residency at Cedars-Sinai Medical Center; she earned her PharmD and BS in Biology at the University of Michigan.

Kallie's advice is: *Your plans will change at some point; use the communication skills you've developed throughout your residency training to navigate the transition. In particular, enlist the support and advice of your mentors and supervisors to help you along the way. Don't be afraid to examine what attracts you to an area of practice. You may find that it helps you adapt to change more easily.*

Dear Pharmacy Colleague,

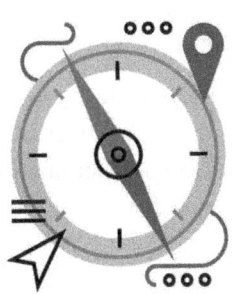

During my first year of pharmacy school, a series of guest speakers spoke to our class and detailed their professional careers. A common theme in their stories was how an unexpected opportunity led them to their current states. I never expected to have a similar story in my own path.

I expected my own career trajectory to plod along in an uneventful fashion. Having decided that I wanted to be a pharmacist while I was in high school, I laid out my plan to accomplish that goal. I planned to attend the University of Michigan for my under-graduate degree—which I did. I planned to stay at the university to attend pharmacy school—which I also did. Thus, after deciding that I wanted to be a pharmacist in high school, the first eight years of my path went exactly according to my plan. While still completing my undergraduate coursework, I was drawn to the world of hospital pharmacy and enticed by the cooperation among various health disciplines. During my pharmacy internship, I discovered the world of emergency medicine and felt I had found my niche. The critical thinking, excitement, and team atmosphere in an emer-gency department (ED) spurred me to take as many critical care and ED rotations as I could throughout my P4 year and select a PGY1 with additional learning opportunities in critical care. Luckily, I found a PGY1 at a program that allowed my husband and me to stay in Michigan.

PGY1 was as challenging as reputed. It only took until late August of my PGY1 for my husband to state, "I hate residency," as I settled on the couch for another evening of reading. Students and preceptors widely acknowledge the challenges of residency, but very little of my (intense) research for PGY1 prepared me for the challenges it would present to my marriage. My husband and I underestimated how the hours and workload of PGY1 would affect our communication and job-sharing responsibilities. We had to find a new equilibrium. One of our solutions was to find ways to more efficiently complete our routine chores—like purchasing a robot vacuum we've affec-tionately named "Geoffrey."

As always seems to happen, once we settled into our new routine to manage the challenges of PGY1, life introduced a new wrinkle. My husband was offered a great career opportunity across the country in sunny Los Angeles. We had talked about moving there so we could be closer to family, but we didn't anticipate the opportunity to come when it did. Although he moved across the country midway through my PGY1, I attended the ASHP Midyear and interviewed for PGY2 residencies. Knowing how difficult PGY1 was, the idea of pursuing a PGY2 seemed crazy. However, I knew that a PGY2 would set me up well for the rest of my career.

The PGY2 programs that interested me spanned the country, and I was prepared to spend additional time away from my family to develop my skills. Despite this, my husband unconditionally supported me in this decision and actively helped me prepare for interviews and settle on my rank list.

As the match drew closer, I envisioned two possible outcomes for my next year: (1) I would match with a great program and grow my skillset as an emergency medicine pharmacist, or (2) I would join my husband in Los Angeles and seek a position at a hospital as an inpatient pharmacist. I was excited about both prospects and ready for the coming change.

When Match Day dawned and I received the email revealing my unmatched state, I switched gears to work toward a staff position in a market where I had no connections. I began consolidating the list of open positions I wanted to pursue in California. One of my mentors had a connection at Cedars-Sinai and offered to reach out and pass along my résumé. The director of pharmacy replied to my mentor and asked if I were interested in a new PGY2 opportunity specializing in transitions of care. Despite completing an ambulatory care student rotation with a transitions of care component, I had not considered it as a possible career choice. Until that point, I had been focused on preparing for a career in emergency medicine or critical care. While I did some self-reflection and considered the new opportunity, I asked my mentors for their advice. During that process, I found out something new about myself. My mentors helped me discover a current of care transitions that wove through my patient care, no matter the setting. As BB King said, *The beautiful thing about learning is nobody can take it away from you,"* and I felt the experience could only help me become a stronger clinician. Ultimately, I decided that the opportunity to learn from pharmacy leaders and become a more balanced practitioner was not something I could pass up.

A few short months after starting my second residency, I discovered I was pregnant. Someone once told me that there is no good time to have a baby, and I responded that there are some points in life that are better than others. I didn't think getting pregnant during PGY2 was one of those "better" times, and starting a family during a residency year certainly changed how I experienced both my pregnancy and my residency rather than if they had happened separately. I knew that my pregnancy would require some adjustments to my year as well as open communication with my preceptors. I told my program director as soon as my husband and I felt comfortable so that we could formulate a plan. I was upfront about my intention to finish residency, when I planned to return after leave, and how I expected to stay on track with projects and assignments. My director had already become a mentor to me, and she continued to support me as I navigated this new challenge. I was fortunate to have a program director and preceptors who understood and helped me achieve my goals.

Having my son has been the most paradigm-shifting experience of my life. I was fortunate to have an easy, healthy pregnancy and baby, and I chose to look at the unavoidable inconveniences as first-hand experience to share with my patients. For instance, I have a much better understanding of how non-pharmacological strategies are not always enough when it comes to acid reflux! I will also admit that the increased challenge of pregnancy paled in comparison to balancing a newborn and residency. I opted to return to work after 6 weeks of leave to complete my final weeks of residency. Once again, I needed a new equilibrium to balance my family and residency obligations. In fact, I found that my new family life has become the greatest motivator to be proactive and complete things in a timely manner while simultaneously making it more difficult to do so.

As my residency drew to a close, I reflected on the experiences I've collected throughout my education. I found the following themes carried me through, which may be helpful as your career begins:

- Derive what interests you about a specialty to the most basic level; it may open up new areas of interest that involve those tenets.

- Open communication—whether with family, mentors, or supervisors—makes new challenges a little more manageable.

- It's not always easy, but plans change, and that's OK.

Pharmacy training and family life can coexist successfully—there are plenty of examples across the country. What helped me the most was the knowledge that my education would make me a better pharmacist, and it would someday allow me to share my passion with my son to help others. Always remember:

- Your plans will change at some point; use the communication skills you've developed throughout your training to navigate the transition.

- In particular, enlist the support and advice of your mentors and supervisors to help you along the way.

- Don't be afraid to examine what attracts you to an area of practice. You may find that it helps you adapt to change more easily.

Kallie

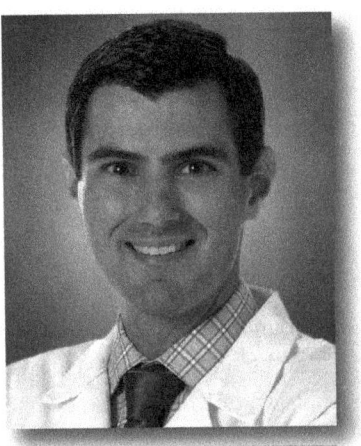

Keith G. Anderson
PharmD, BCPS

Making the Tough Training and Career Decisions

Keith, who comes from a small town and from a family with a limited healthcare background, has leveraged a residency to work clinically at one of the largest healthcare organizations in the country. This letter, describing his experiences, reflects many of the decisions facing young pharmacy students today. We are fortunate to have him in health-system pharmacy as the profession is in good hands for the future.

Keith is currently Inpatient Nursing Unit-Based Pharmacist at Cleveland Clinic (Heart and Vascular Institute), Ohio. He completed the postgraduate year 1 (PGY1) pharmacy practice residency at the Cleveland Clinic. Keith received his PharmD from Ohio Northern University, Ada.

Keith's advice is: *When you encounter an inspirational moment in your personal or professional life, reflect on your next steps to build on that experience. At times the path may seem hidden, but from my experience each decision you make will provide more clarity.*

Dear Pharmacy Colleague,

Early in your career you are faced with many tough decisions, and at times, the possibility of making the wrong choice can feel terrifying. Without a doubt, you've already made at

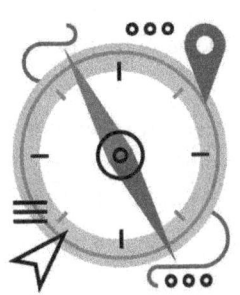

least several big decisions that have shaped your life: pursuing higher education, selecting a university, choosing a major, and perhaps even plotting out your post-graduation career plans. In making these decisions, you have already begun shaping the path your professional and personal life will take. *Allow me to share a word of advice*—don't let this scare you; every decision will provide new opportunities to learn, grow, and pursue the career you desire. Furthermore, the inspiration to make these tough decisions often comes when you least expect it or from the most surprising places. Let me share how experiences and people shaped some of the biggest decisions thus far early in my career, including my decision to pursue a residency.

Because I grew up in a small Ohio town to a family with a limited healthcare experience, my decision to pursue pharmacy began with little first-hand information. My only knowledge of the profession was gleaned from our local retail pharmacist. Undeterred by the uncertainty, I decided to pursue a degree in pharmacy given its strong foundation in math and science, united with the desire to help others. It turned out to be one of my best decisions. The thought of attending a large university in a big town terrified me, so I enrolled in the pharmacy program at Ohio Northern University, a small Division III school in rural western Ohio. I couldn't have been further removed or more unfamiliar with the field of clinical inpatient pharmacy and could not even imagine that's where I would end up six years later. However, during my first year of college, I took an elective class. Pharmacy alumni came in as guest lecturers to describe their careers from a variety of different fields within pharmacy. To this day, I distinctly remember a pharmacist coming to our small classroom and describing her role as a cardiology clinical specialist at the Cleveland Clinic. I was fascinated and intrigued by the thought of working in a hospital as part of a collaborative medical team, making drug therapy recommendations.

When you encounter an inspirational moment in your personal or professional life, reflect on your next steps to build upon that experience. At times the path may seem hidden, but from my experience each decision you make will provide more clarity. After that exposure to the practice of a clinical pharmacist, I began planning my own path to pursue such a career. I started with an internship at a local retail pharmacy. Two years later, I leveraged that professional experience into obtaining an internship at a small regional hospital. I also began working with one of my professors on a research project aimed at discovering compounds to target a novel antimicrobial enzyme utilizing molecular modeling. These opportunities were not only fulfilling, but also served to build my resume when I later decided to pursue a residency. Having been through both sides of the residency-ranking process and job interviews, there is no single blueprint that identifies the perfect candidate. However, previous experiences in any number of forms will help to distinguish you from other candidates and also provide the opportunity for you to reflect on how they have shaped and prepared you for the position you are pursuing.

My experiences during pharmacy school introduced me to three key mentors who were instrumental in shaping my career. The *first* was a manager during my internship at the local retail pharmacy. It was my first job experience of any kind in the field of pharmacy. From him, I learned to always put the well-being and safety of patients first. The *second* was the professor at Ohio Northern with whom I worked on the aforementioned research project. He encouraged me to pursue my own ideas and was the first person to help me truly foster a sense of independence. The *third* mentor was the clinical pharmacist who visited our classroom. In addition to being the first person to expose me to a career in clinical pharmacy, she also served as my preceptor on an advanced pharmacy practice experience (APPE) rotation. She became a role model as to how a clinical pharmacist should practice and demonstrated the value a good preceptor can have in shaping the experience of learners.

All three mentors were invaluable to my career in other critical ways, including serving as references. I cannot overemphasize the importance of having a mentor at different points in your educational experiences and career. They can be vital in fostering your professional growth because of their professional and personal experiences. When it is time to make tough decisions, they can also provide sage advice or the inspiration to take a chance.

DIFFICULT DECISIONS

The first difficult decision I encountered when finishing pharmacy school was how to choose a residency program. Various factors may influence your decision: *How big is the hospital? Where is it located? How many co-residents will you have? Does the hospital offer any PGY2 residencies and the opportunity to early commit?* I interviewed with residency programs of different sizes, in different states, with different opportunities. Ultimately, the most important factor was how I saw myself fitting in with the culture of the program. This is a difficult concept to describe and was more of a gut-feeling from my interaction during interviews with the preceptors and current residents, and whether I could see myself as a resident at that program. From the uncertainty in deciding how to rank different residency sites, to what feels like an excruciating wait for Match Day to arrive (in reality it is just a couple of weeks!) and the anxiety of receiving the match results email, the entire ASHP match process can be a roller coaster of emotions, culminating in the excitement of finding out the results. To this day, one of my favorite movie quotes still comes from Tom Hanks in the Academy Award winning film *Forest Gump*: "*Mama always said life was like a box of chocolates. You never know what you're gonna get.*" No single day has better captured this sentiment than how I felt on Match Day for my PGY1 pharmacy practice residency. My journey would lead me to matching with the Cleveland Clinic, a 1400-bed hospital where I would have fifteen other co-residents. In terms of size and scope, it was a far cry from my small rural university. However, I was confident when ranking the Cleveland Clinic based on my experiences there on APPE rotations and how I felt my personality would mix with the culture of the program.

Benefits of Residency Experiences. My experiences during residency are ones I will never forget. I learned more than I could possibly imagine from some truly brilliant preceptors and became more confident giving presentations. (Public speaking has always been a fear of mine!) More importantly, the preceptors helped refine my critical thinking skills, something I continue to be thankful for to this day. Beyond the learning experience, I developed close friendships with my co-residents who have moved on to positions all across the country and done remarkable things in their early careers. I often hear the saying *"pharmacy is a small world,"* and I have found this to be true. Between the preceptors, co-residents, and others you meet along the way, residency offers a wonderful networking opportunity that can provide dividends the rest of your career.

MORE CAREER DECISIONS

Despite the long hours, it is also an experience that will fly by. Before I realized, it was time to make a decision about pursuing a PGY2 residency. I completed several critical care rotations early in my residency year and considered pursing a PGY2 in this specialty even though I knew cardiology was my true passion. All of my fellow PGY1 co-residents had made the decision to pursue PGY2 residencies, including several who early committed. I felt an internal pressure to follow the same path and even completed interviews with some programs. Meanwhile, my intuition was telling me it didn't feel like the right decision. I didn't feel the same passion or sense of belonging at those programs. After discussions with my residency program director who provided amazing support on a difficult decision, I withdrew before the match.

I suppose my career may have taken a very different turn had I decided to go through with the match for a PGY2 critical care residency. Looking back, I have absolutely no regrets. I had the good fortune to be hired upon completion of my PGY1 residency into a nursing unit-based pharmacist position at the Cleveland Clinic. When I reflect on why the Cleveland Clinic was the right decision for me, it all clicks when I read the values of our department: *"Enabling and empowering each individual in the Department of Pharmacy to make valuable contributions to patient-focused care, teaching, and research activities."*

These values match so perfectly with the ideals the three mentors instilled in me: always put patients first, develop your independence to pursue your own ideas, and be a preceptor and role model to prepare the next generation of pharmacists.

Things have a funny way of coming full circle. All of the experiences I had along the way allowed me to fulfill the idea I had during my first year of pharmacy school— to work in a hospital as part of a collaborative medical team making drug therapy recommendations. As for the clinical pharmacist who inspired me to pursue such a career, I am fortunate to still call her a role-model, mentor, and now co-worker. I feel blessed to have the opportunity to work at one of the top hospitals in the nation, collaborating with cardiology and vascular surgery teams, and precepting some of the brilliant future pharmacists.

There are plenty of tough decisions you will have to make in your career. Remember to reflect on the people and experiences that provide the inspiration to take the next step. Behind every decision awaits a new opportunity.

Keith

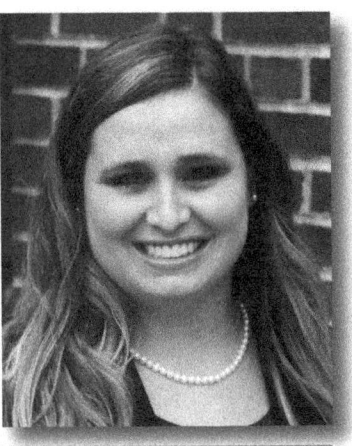

Ali Lloyd Baker
PharmD, MS

Finding Your Anchors in a Sea of Change

Ali's mission statement is to be a leader worth following and, given her letter, she is well on her way. You will find that she is very nimble and resilient because of the challenges she successfully handled during her two-year residency. She indicates that her best learning came from her mistakes, not her successes.

Ali is currently Pharmacy System Manager, Wake Forest Baptist Health, Winston-Salem, North Carolina. She completed a postgraduate year 1 (PGY1) accredited pharmacy practice residency and accredited PGY2 health-system pharmacy administration residency at Wake Forest Baptist Health, having received her MS from the University of North Carolina, Chapel Hill and her PharmD from Samford University, McWhorter School of Pharmacy, in Birmingham, Alabama.

Ali's advice is: ***Learning to adapt in an environment of constant change is the most important principle I learned during my health-system pharmacy administration residency.***

Dear Pharmacy Colleague,

> The pessimist complains about the wind;
> the optimist expects it to change;
> the realist adjusts the sails.
> —William Arthur Ward

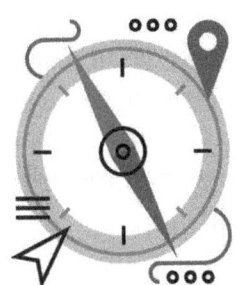

Learning to adapt in an environment of constant change is the most important principle I learned during my health-system pharmacy administration (HSPA) residency. To begin, I'd like to tell you a little about my experience at ASHP's Midyear Clinical Meeting and the Personnel Placement Service (PPS) process. After meeting with an almost-overwhelming fifteen programs during PPS and meeting many more at the Showcase, a few programs quickly rose to the top of my list. On Match Day, I learned I was placed with Wake Forest Baptist Health, my #1 choice. The director, also my future residency program director, said in a text message, "We could not be more excited to see that you have matched with us! Congratulations on a successful match; you are entering into a fantastic world within pharmacy, and we are going to have a blast!" I still have the text saved on my phone. Initially, that was a strong indication to me that my mentor was dedicated and excited to lead me as a resident.

Several months went by with preparation for a move to North Carolina, leaving a city that had been my home away from home for six years and starting my professional career. I instinctively knew that residency was going to be different from fourth-year rotations; but even so, I was dedicated to this decision and this leadership team. With every email or letter from Wake Forest, I reinvested in my commitment.

Four weeks before residency was scheduled to begin, I received a call from a current HSPA resident at Wake Forest who informed me that there was a change of leadership within the pharmacy department. The director and residency program director who recruited me no longer worked there. Initially, I was in disbelief. The person I had begun to connect to would not be there. At that time, it was undetermined who would be leading the HSPA residency. It was a lot to consider for a new resident entering a program.

Within the first 12 months of my residency, I experienced three leadership transitions. The first leader made a great first impression as a strong recruiter, but was not there to manage my initial entrance. The second leader doubted my ability and fit with the program. But the third leader embraced me as my mentor and helped me grow far beyond my expectations.

I would like to offer some advice learned from how I dealt with these circumstances. We all know that change is inevitable. That doesn't mean we are ready for it. The more mature we are in our careers, the better equipped we are to handle change. But as a resident, especially a HSPA resident, I was required to take a crash course on change management. This required me to find my personal anchors to steady me as I rode out the sea of change. I would like to share those anchors in hopes that it will be valuable to future residents riding the same waves!

The Anchor of Trust—*Building a reputation of trust is essential.* When management issues are shared with you, you must keep them confidential and not share them. This is no longer a college campus where gossip is recreational. This takes maturity. You must establish trustworthiness with the management team and with your fellow residents.

This is particularly challenging when you feel caught between a member of the management team and a fellow resident. For example, I was privy to information related to a new leader joining the team weeks before the department was informed. It is difficult when your residents ask you for information you are not able to provide. When this occurred, I took the open approach by sharing that the department will be updated as soon as possible.

I'm sure you've heard the phrase, "Trust is very difficult to gain, and easy to lose." And in residency, when you are under the microscope, that is exponentially true. Navigating situations where you work with many preceptors, and in my experience, many direct supervisors, knowing who to trust and when to trust is key. In the beginning, it is reasonable to make mistakes, but learning from those mistakes and moving forward as a trustworthy person is what is important and essential for your success.

The Anchor of Resiliency—*You must learn to rebound.* Many days, things do not go as planned. There will be conflict and disappointment. As a young professional, it is likely you will want to always be successful. That is not realistic. You will be given negative or "constructive" feedback. What you do with the feedback is important. Do you become offended? Are you defensive or hurt? Does it motivate you or discourage you? The hardest lessons in life are generally learned from our mistakes, not our successes. You must pick yourself up and keep going.

I quickly learned that feedback does not come from one direction (or one person) but from every direction. This is one of the most important skills that residency will teach you.

At one point in my residency, the two most influential people in my residency, my residency program director and my advisor, both questioned my intentions and my fit within the program. This was extremely tough for me to hear. It was even more difficult for me to get on a plane the next day to recruit the next HSPA class at ASHP's Midyear Clinical Meeting. What I learned from that experience is that in all circumstances, find your anchor of resiliency. It's crucial for you in times when others doubt your ability or skillset. Luckily, I was able to demonstrate my resiliency in residency; but to be honest, it would have been much easier to quit. But I didn't sign up for residency just to give up.

Resiliency is the anchor I held on to the most during residency. I hope it is not the same for you; however, know that once you navigate through the tough situation, people will either remember that you persevered or will not realize that you survived challenging circumstances.

The Anchor of Adaptability—*Things change.* Be able to adapt to change. Throughout my second year, while on administration-focused rotations, five primary preceptors on the leadership team left for other opportunities. Losing half the leadership team was difficult, created uncertainty, and offered opportunities with responsibilities that otherwise would not have been available.

Upon reflection, I believe that learning to roll with the punches (or any other pun you want to insert here) is without question a valuable lesson learned during residency. All in all, I watched as ten department leaders left. It's interesting to reflect back on how the department adapted to these changes, and especially how it affected us.

The Anchor of Adding Value—*You should never focus on meeting expectations.* Always strive to go beyond what is requested, such as filling in where needed or volunteering.

Throughout the leadership changes, it took me a while to gain the perspective that I had become a constant presence for the frontline staff. My staffing area throughout my two-year residency was our Central Pharmacy. I knew all the staff, and they knew me. When I started, I was new but eager to learn. I consistently worked weekend staffing assignments and came back on Monday with several recommendations for improvement. Additionally, I became a good listener and sounding board for the staff. I believe it was simply my presence in the area, working alongside pharmacists and technicians that connected us. I took their concerns seriously and would escalate or run interference when needed. Once I realized I had become their constant, I was able to help them handle the changes by providing perspective.

Adding value can look different in various situations. For me, I added value the most by being present and caring for others dealing with the uncertainty of our leadership changes. Often, I wouldn't have any answers, but my consistency and constant presence added value.

The Anchor of Humility—*You should strive to be a servant leader to your team.* This means understanding the importance of focusing on the department's success before your own individual success. To achieve this, you try to lift others up before yourself, practice humility, avoid grabbing the glory, and sincerely care about others by placing their needs before your own.

A large snowstorm hit North Carolina during my second year of residency. We began to plan for the impending storm. I was scheduled to be our staffing coordinator on-call, which meant I would be responsible for managing all the call-outs and other staffing issues that week. Even with much preplanning, several staff members were unable to arrive for their scheduled shifts that weekend so I had to manage/juggle the available staff with work areas. All in all, even with 10 inches of snow, we were able to make it through the weekend with minimal issues. The following week at many leadership meetings, I was recognized for my skills and abilities throughout the weekend: understanding who can work in which areas and contacting others to be available in advance, etc. In my mind, the real heroes were the pharmacists and technicians who faced the snowstorm to be present for work, making sure all the shifts were properly covered.

In retrospect, I wish I could have felt more proud in that moment instead of embarrassed by the recognition. There are many instances where I should have acted with more humility—we all have those moments. However, the message I want to share is to be proud of the work you complete and continue to be humble at the same time.

The good news is that riding the sea of change paid off for me. During my second year of residency, our hospital recruited a highly regarded chief pharmacy officer who has steadied the ship with a vision of enhanced pharmacy operations. I was fortunate to be hired as a systems manager with staff management responsibilities and dynamic growth initiatives.

The truth is these principles, or anchors, stay with me in my professional advancement. What I've learned is that healthcare and its management is rapidly evolving. With a strong team and a commitment to trust, resiliency, adaptability, value, and humility, you will be well prepared to adjust your sails toward success and career fulfillment.

Wishing you smooth sailing,

Ali

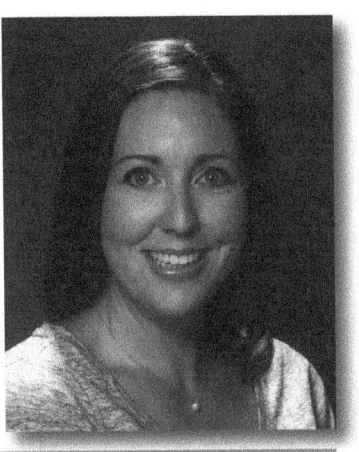

Margeaux (Maggie) Byrd
PharmD

Invest in Your Future, Dive in, and Take the Risk

Maggie demonstrates her passion and enthusiasm for the pharmacy profession, and during her residency she wanted to make a difference. This fit well with her project choice, implementing a Transitions of Care pharmacist position for the hospital. Maggie is outgoing and approachable, and she connects well with her patients and members of the healthcare team. She has a strong commitment to patient care and balances her career and family life well.

Maggie is currently Clinical Pharmacist, MultiCare Auburn Medical Center, Washington. Maggie completed her accredited postgraduate year 1 (PGY1) residency at MultiCare Good Samaritan Hospital, Puyallup, Washington and received her PharmD degree at the University of Montana, Missoula. Maggie also received her BA degree at Carroll College, Helena, Montana with a double major in chemistry and psychology.

Maggie's advice is: *A residency is an opportunity to refine your professional self. It is a symbiotic investment—between you and your site. If you want it, go for it. Dive in and take the risk—it will be worth it.*

Dear Pharmacy Colleague,

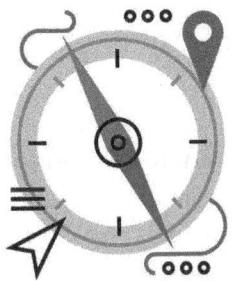

The decision to pursue a residency has been one my greatest accomplishments. It was personally driven, which resulted in clinical and individual growth. I hope a glimpse into my journey offers some guidance for yours.

IF YOU WANT IT, GO FOR IT

As a former bartender, those around me can attest that my strengths involve people skills. During pharmacy school, I was that student in class who made her morning rounds with each classmate, checking in, and offering a humiliating story about myself with the satisfaction of knowing I made someone smile. A procrastinator, still to this day, my energy was instinctively directed toward building relationships, not memorizing text books and analyzing clinical studies. I held officer positions in almost every club. In addition to my extracurricular activities, I worked 1 or 2 jobs, started school with a newborn, and thought it was a great idea to have another baby during my third year. My husband traveled for work, so as you can imagine, I slept very little during pharmacy school. I share this background of juggling children, school, jobs, and extracurricular activities because when the idea of pursuing a residency was presented, you can understand why I avoided it.

I have always known the value of a pharmacy residency. Working at hospitals with residents, and witnessing close friends take on this endeavor, I saw their amazing transformation to becoming confident and strong clinical pharmacists; however, I also saw their struggles. I heard stories of late nights, challenging working environments, never-ending projects, lack of a social life, and less than appealing salaries. If you asked me if I was going to do a residency, I hesitated. I desired to be the clinical pharmacist my friends were becoming, however; I doubted if I could match, and with two kids and my husband starting his career, I had more than myself to think about. Besides, my strong interpersonal skills were not reflected on my exam scores, and I was already beginning to feel some burnout after pushing myself so hard during pharmacy school. So, I asked myself: Was I residency material?

The answer: **Yes.**

The most important quality for pursuing a residency is a desire to be in one. Do not let rumors, statistics, or fear persuade you from residency. Grades, extracurricular activities, and reputations are all important, but are all meaningless unless you have desire. A residency should not be a check box on your resume. I know many former residents have viewed it as such, and in some moments I did as well. However, a residency is an opportunity to refine your professional self. It is a symbiotic investment— between you and your site. If you want it, go for it.

FINDING YOUR MATCH

Applying for a residency is a challenging process and can be very stressful at times. With my lingering hesitation, I took the risk and flew to ASHP's Midyear Meeting to investigate residencies. I arrived completely unprepared and drowned in the sea of business suits. Every person I met had pearls of wisdom for me. I was told what to wear, what to say and how to say it, which residencies to look at, how to get "in" with directors, and so much more. All I could hear was what everyone else was saying, and I no longer knew what I wanted or how to find it. While staring at my friend's meticulously organized residency list, I decided to listen to my own voice.

This was the pivotal point in my residency journey—I chose to reflect on what I wanted in a residency. All accredited residencies must have certain core rotations and meet standards. I recommend investigating in what sites have to offer that makes them different or stand out from other programs. For me, I wanted a strong emergency department and a site that was well-established. I was never committed to a particular area of pharmacy, so I searched for a site that offered a variety of rotations. Next, I valued work environment. When I visited, talked, and interviewed with different sites, I always asked if co-workers socialized outside of work. This was crucial to me because it was a sign people enjoyed each other in and outside the workplace. Interacting with people is important to me, so I focused on applying to residencies that shared my core values and invested in the residents. Finally, I had children; location was important to me. Although I did apply to a couple sites across the country, I valued my husband's input. If I was going to do a residency, I needed all the support possible.

We all have unique circumstances, and mine was my family. The more I talked with other students, the more I did not feel alone. Very few have the option to apply wherever they want without considerations for extenuating situations, be it family, spouse, or private hardships. Do not feel alone or discouraged if you are limited to where you can apply.

In all, I interviewed at seven different residency sites. Each interview had similarities such as some clinical skills component, a required presentation, and one-on-one interviews. Sometimes I was caught off guard with a question or went blank during a clinical question; however, these are secretly the best moments to shine. If you do not know the answer, do not lie or make it up. Simply explain what you would do in the situation. Always be honest and market your strengths. Come prepared, refreshed, and dressed professionally. Practice interview questions with friends, know your strengths and weaknesses, and relax. And guess what? If you are not a good match with a site, that is OK! The interview is an opportunity for the site to know you beyond your application and for you to get a glimpse of the site and people first hand.

Next step was to rank my sites and pray. For me, waiting was almost the worst part. My joy of matching was dampened when I saw a few of my classmates not match. Many of them, to this day, would have been a far better resident than me. Did they present themselves poorly in an interview? Were their grades worse than I thought? Did they limit themselves too much? As these questions flooded my mind, I can only imagine their disappointment. Unfortunately, there is risk when applying for a residency and not everyone matches. If you do not match, you are not alone. Hindsight can be beneficial, but sometimes it's as simple as tough competition and how the algorithm of the match determined your fate. My co-resident did not match his first attempt. He worked in the community for the following year and reapplied. Because he was already a practicing pharmacist when we met, he was a huge support in helping me study for my exams. He was an amazing resident, and I deeply admire his commitment to pursue a residency. He continued to follow his passion, and successfully matched to a second-year program—first time around.

IT GOES BY FAST

The year of residency challenged me in many ways. I was blessed to have matched with a program that did more than teach me, they invested in my professional development and personal growth—which is exactly what I wanted. This does not mean it was an easy year. I worked long days, often frustrated and overwhelmed, missed out on family events, and sometimes found myself wondering what my life would have been without doing a residency. However, as I sit here typing this letter, I am incredibly proud of surviving my residency year and amazed how far I have come as a clinical pharmacist. I gained the confidence and clinical thinking skills needed to optimize patient care. More importantly, I grew as a person and learned more about myself.

How did I survive? Relationships and communication. You are not stranded on an island like in an episode of Survivor. It is a single year focused on clinical refinement with occasional growing pains. Preceptors and directors want you to be successful. Speak up if you need help. They will not know what you need unless you tell them. Remember they are juggling many demands as well. Do not forget to laugh with your preceptors, take humility in acknowledging you do not know something, be honest about your mistakes, and appreciate the journey.

Finally, take the time to build relationships with your co-resident(s). I only had one co-resident, and I do not think we could have been more opposite—different backgrounds, cultures, strengths, and even humor. We did not instantly connect. But the more we reached out to each other, sharing our stories, the closer we became. We made efforts to eat lunch together, attend social events, and, occasionally, secretly vent our frustrations. Because it was just the two of us, we made an effort to associate with a larger residency program within the same healthcare system. The relationships you build during this year are unique and amazing. Put forth the effort with co-residents; you will not regret it.

FINDING YOUR NEXT STEP

It can be difficult to comprehend life post-residency because residency is full of uncertainties. During residency, my mind was focused on the present, not the future. Although definite decisions are not necessary early on, keep the future in mind. If you are considering a second-year residency, plan your rotations accordingly. For example, if you want to specialize in oncology in a PGY2, make sure you have an oncology rotation completed before applications are due. I was fortunate to have a director who initiated these conversations, so speak up if these are not addressed. Also, there are many opportunities throughout the year to make connections for jobs after residencies. Once again, make relationships and market yourself throughout your residency. However, do not let the stress about what will happen after residency derail you from your current commitment. My site hired many former residents; however, when I graduated, my director was unable to offer a full-time position which I needed with my piling debt and outrageous daycare costs. She connected me with another director at a nearby hospital within the same healthcare system in which I got a full-time clinical pharmacist position.

Currently, I am in my first-year post-residency. I can say without hesitation, my residency prepared me to be a confident and knowledgeable member of the healthcare team. When I receive calls from physicians and nurses, I am able to ask important clinical questions and help direct medical decisions to benefit the patient and team. My residency gave me the tools to be successful when triaging drug shortages, handle intense moments such as codes, and answer challenging questions. It inspired me to be part of the ever-changing healthcare environment and helped me realize that becoming a clinical pharmacist is a lifelong journey, with continual opportunities to grow.

Choosing to do a residency is a personal choice. Can you be a great pharmacist without doing a residency? Yes, of course. Can you be happy without doing a residency? Yes. Will your colleagues respect you if you do *not* do a residency? Yes. If timing is not right or you have no interest in residency, that is OK too.

However, if you want it, go for it. Invest in your future, dive in, and take the risk—it will be worth it.

Sincerely,

Maggie

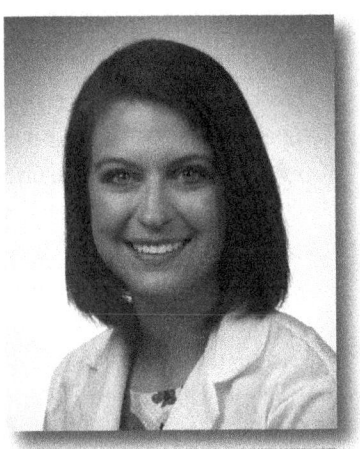

Lindsey Coval Cooper
PharmD

Maximizing Feedback and Being the Chief Resident

You will find Lindsey is a very insightful person who seeks to learn from all her experiences. She is good at applying learning from non-pharmacy settings to her pharmacy practice. In addition to her patients, Lindsey is attuned to her healthcare workers' understanding of how each person's role is essential for excellent patient care.

Lindsey is currently a Critical Care Clinical Pharmacist at Palmetto Health Richland, Columbia, South Carolina. She completed her postgraduate year 1 (PGY1) pharmacy practice residency and PGY2 critical care pharmacy residency at Palmetto Health. Lindsey received her PharmD from the Wilkes University Nesbitt School of Pharmacy, Pennsylvania.

Lindsey's advice is: **For times when you are not sure how to take the feedback or what to do with it, remember that feedback is truly a gift to be thankful for; then write it down to return to later.**

Dear Pharmacy Colleague,

As I was preparing for residency, most of the tips I got entailed how to stay organized and manage my time. Although each of those tips was incredibly helpful, three pieces

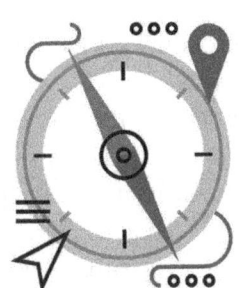

of advice in particular helped me during my PGY1 and PGY2 residencies and transitioning into being a critical care pharmacist: everyone is a cog in the wheel, the platinum rule, and the importance of feedback.

A Cog in the Wheel. The first piece of advice is that every person is a cog in a wheel regardless of title, training, or education. When I was a student, one of my preceptors gave me that advice. He said that when people start letting titles and training become more important than taking care of patients, they unintentionally start to remove cogs from the wheel. As you can imagine, if a wheel is missing—even one cog—it does not turn properly; but remove multiple cogs, and it just stops. Thus, every cog becomes equally important. Many student pharmacists worked as technicians, and now that they have their pharmacy license, they will perform a new job with new duties. Those who are completing residencies will learn operations functions, but may ultimately end up working as decentralized clinical pharmacists. The acknowledgment that every position is equally important in helping a patient will afford the resident not just a more pleasant experience and a better ability to work with others, but also will open the door to truly learn how each job affects the patient and how the resident can be more impactful to the patient.

This concept was further solidified during one of my emergency medicine residency rotations in which my preceptor said "A lot of times it's all hands on deck up here. I am not above doing anything for a patient if it is what needs to be done (without exceeding the limits of my license, of course)." If that meant gathering a patient's belongings from the trauma bay or getting a patient a drink, that is what our role was at that time. As I transitioned from a resident to a full-time pharmacist, I realized that willingness to jump in when needed makes the wheel turn more efficiently, and other members of the team recognize and are grateful. Frequently, an urgent procedure must be done at the bedside in the intensive care unit (ICU) that does not require medications aside from those already ordered. My role in these situations is to help the patient's family find the waiting room, help the nurses quickly gather supplies, or answer the phone for the nurse. Many times it may not seem like there is anything I can do, but a simple "Is there anything I can do for you right now?" to any member of the team often reveals even something small that they would appreciate help with.

The Platinum Rule. *The second piece of advice is to follow the platinum rule as opposed to the golden rule.* One of my previous supervisors who did a great deal of leadership training and reading often taught this concept authored by Dr. Tony Allesandra. We all know the golden rule is something to the effect of *"Treat others the way* ***YOU*** *want to be treated."* The platinum rule goes further—*"Treat others the way* ***THEY*** *want to be treated."* It obviously takes more effort to follow the platinum rule considering it requires getting to know the people you are working with and even those you work with infrequently. The effort pays off, though. On one of my first shifts in the intravenous (IV) room as a resident, I was working with two technicians who I had not trained with. I quickly learned that each technician accomplished tasks very differently. During a busy time, I asked if there was anything I could do to help them. One technician said that he could handle it and showed that he took great ownership in his work, while the other technician said she could handle it but would be grateful for any help. Going forward, I handled busy periods differently for the two. For the first technician, I never stopped offering to help, but always acknowledged that I knew he would prefer to take care of all of his tasks by himself. For the second technician, if we were backed up, I would take some of the printed labels and take care of them, because I knew she was OK with it. This seems like something incredibly simple, but truthfully, my gut reaction when it is busy is to just jump in and start helping get things done. Depending on the person, if I had done that, I could have left the first technician feeling like I did not think he was capable of the work or that I thought I could do it faster. Not helping the second technician may have left her feeling that I did not care that we were backed up or that I did not think it was my job to make IVs. Neither would have made for a good working relationship or help me build a rapport with either technician.

Feedback. The third piece of advice that I am incredibly grateful to have received during my second rotation of residency is that feedback is a gift. This advice came at a time when I was receiving evaluations for my first rotation, feedback on my research protocol for institutional review board (IRB) submission, and beginning to work the weekend clinical rotation. At times, it seemed like one piece of feedback was the exact opposite of another I had received. *How was I supposed to take the feedback and incorporate it into my projects or practice?* The amount of feedback you get can become overwhelming. Luckily, my preceptor reminded me that all of it is important even if it is conflicting. You should be grateful for the opportunity to have so many people helping to make you a better practitioner. Another preceptor always liked to remind her residents that residency would be the last time they will receive this much feedback or have someone else evaluating them so closely. Sorting through feedback can be difficult, and depending on what it is and how it was given, it can have some emotion tied to it, good or bad. For times when you are not sure how to take the feedback or what to do with it, remember that it is truly a gift. Be thankful for it, but write it down to return to later.

When you return to that feedback, there are multiple questions you can ask yourself: *What does the feedback actually pertain to? Does it conflict with other feedback you have received; if so, how? Is the feedback generalizable or specific to a particular project or rotation? How can the feedback be incorporated going forward?* There are a plethora of questions you could ask, but these are a good start. In addition to all the clinical knowledge you will learn during residency, learning how to really take and process feedback is actually a skill you will learn, too.

An example of a time when I had to return to feedback was during one of my major residency projects. The feedback was geared toward a completely different direction than I had taken on in my project, and there were multiple preceptors' inputs. Because I had put so much work into the project, there was obviously some emotion tied to it. At first, I was not sure what exactly to do with all of the feedback, as it initially seemed

I needed to start over. So, I wrote it all down and came back to it a couple of days later. I realized that there were actually only a few things to address. I just needed to sort through the multiple preceptors' feedback, which led me to find that most of it was somewhat similar and only pertained to a few aspects of the project. I still had some conflicting feedback that I had to return to and mull over that was then sorted out in discussions. In the end, I was glad I took the time to gather my thoughts, sort through everything, and not try to start from scratch. In reviewing the feedback, it boiled down to just a few changes and further investigation. The feedback taught me how to really look at the intricacies and rare situations in the formulary review process, and helped me think through the essential questions to ensure appropriate utilization of medications (for such a small proportion of patients with such a significant disease burden). Much of that project's feedback can and will be incorporated into my future formulary review projects.

Not only did all this advice help me during residency and even now in my current job, but it also helped me in my role as chief resident during my PGY2 residency. As chief resident, some of my responsibilities included organizing and preparing for the ASHP Midyear Meeting and residency conference, facilitating group outings, and serving as a liaison between the residents and the Residency Advisory Committee. Sharing my experiences with the PGY1 residents and learning from the things that worked to make the year go smoothly as well as what I would do differently were certainly important in my experiences as the chief resident.

What it really meant to me to be chief resident was just being available for the residents and become comfortable with available resources. In my opinion, my biggest responsibility was helping the residents to navigate and recognize when looking into resources might be beneficial. Some questions just needed a quick answer—where to find something, how to format a presentation, etc. But, for questions such as those pertaining to particular topic areas or for career advice, it was essential for me to know who the appropriate expert in a particular area so I could direct the resident.

For those programs with chief residents, I would encourage residents to truly use them as a resource and as another person to bounce ideas off of. I would also encourage anyone who has the opportunity to serve as chief resident for their residency class to take it. There are obviously responsibilities in addition to your residency responsibilities, but what you gain is worth it. I certainly learned what resources are available and how to find them. I gained a wealth of knowledge about our organization and history of our residency from the Residency Advisory Committee. Whether you are the chief resident or not, you can learn a lot from your co-residents in how each of you accomplishes goals and handles challenges.

During your residency, remember that every person is a cog in the wheel, concentrate on following the platinum rule by getting to know your co-workers, and work hard to distinguish types of feedback. Hopefully you will find these pieces of advice as helpful as I did to quickly form relationships and integrate them into your teams at work.

Lindsey

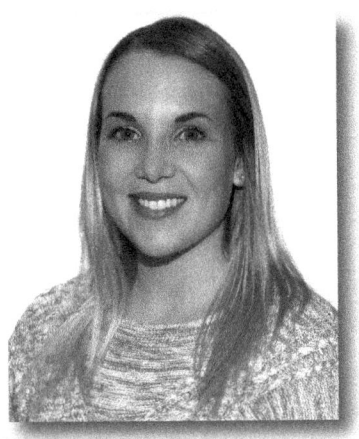

Brienne Costigan
PharmD

Achieve Your Goals through Planning, Persistence, and Maintaining Your Vision

Brienne describes her methodical process for achieving almost all the goals of her career in sequence. Then she experienced a major disappointment—the postgraduate year 2 (PGY2) match. However, with her career goal still intact, she relates how she overcame a major disappointment to achieve her success.

Brienne is currently a Clinical Pharmacist–Pediatrics, at the Floating Hospital for Children at Tufts Medical Center, Boston, Massachusetts. She received her PharmD at the University of Connecticut School of Pharmacy and completed her PGY1 residency at Tufts Medical Center, Boston, Massachusetts.

Brienne's advice is: **Don't let an unexpected setback in your career path prevent you from pursuing and achieving your professional goals and dreams.**

Dear Pharmacy Colleague,

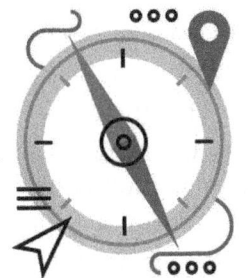

From the time I was 16 years old, I knew that I wanted to become a pharmacist. I excelled in math and the sciences in high school, making a healthcare profession highly suggested by teachers and guidance counselors. Pharmacists were in demand at the time, and family members urged me to consider the profession. I decided to find out for myself whether a career in pharmacy was right for me.

My neighbor was a pharmacist and the owner of an independent pharmacy passed down from her father. She allowed me to shadow her and observe a typical work day. Her knowledge of pharmacology to fill prescriptions and counsel patients on their medications was highly impressive to me. Her personal connection with every patient was admirable. I left her pharmacy that day knowing this was the right career path.

During school breaks at the University of Connecticut, I worked as a paraprofessional for a nonprofit organization providing educational services to children with developmental delays. This unique work experience sparked my passion for working with children, and it was then I realized that I wanted to specialize in the pediatric population.

My introductory pharmacy practice experience (IPPE) gave me insight into the various practice settings. I completed my community experience at my neighbor's pharmacy. My institutional experience was at a hospital, which I enjoyed so much that I decided to stay on as an intern when they offered me a job. This educational experience got me interested in pursuing a residency. I rounded with the clinical pharmacists and was extremely impressed by their involvement in patient care. I loved learning the operational component of pharmacy and understanding the full process of how a medication gets to the patient's bedside from the point of order entry. I knew I was meant to work in a hospital setting.

RESIDENCY PROGRAM DECISIONS

I decided to apply to PGY1 residency programs during my P4 year. I applied to a combination of pediatric specific and general pharmacy practice PGY1 programs. The general pharmacy practice programs all had a required rotation in pediatrics. I wanted to have a solid pediatric foundation that I could potentially expand on by completing a PGY2 specializing in pediatrics. After interviewing at several programs, I decided to rank the general pharmacy practice PGY1 programs at the top of my list. My ultimate goal upon completing a PGY1 program was to become a well-rounded, competent, and confident general practitioner. I felt that I still had so much more to learn about adult medicine, and I didn't want my rotations as a P4 pharmacy student to be my last experience working with adults.

Match Day came, and I was thrilled to find out that I would be going back home to Massachusetts after matching at Tufts Medical Center in Boston. During my PGY1, I completed rotations in five core areas: pediatrics, cancer care, critical care, ambulatory care, and medicine/surgery. My program director gave me the opportunity to have my pediatric rotation block first because he knew this was my area of interest. Taking advantage of this opportunity gave me a great deal of exposure to providing care for this patient population before ASHP's Midyear Clinical Meeting, when I would have to decide whether or not pursuing a PGY2 in pediatrics was right for me. My pediatric rotation experience confirmed what I already knew—I loved working with children and that pursuing a PGY2 in pediatrics was the next step in my career.

I attended the Midyear Meeting and had fourteen interviews with the various pediatric PGY2 programs that I was interested in through Personnel Placement Service. After talking to many amazing program directors and residents to learn more about why their program would be a good fit for me, and for financial reasons, I decided to narrow my list down to five programs. I completed my applications in PhORCAS and hit submit! I was pleased to accept three interviews for PGY2 programs.

January and February were a blur. Between fulfilling current PGY1 responsibilities, including interviewing the next Tufts residency class and traveling to my own PGY2 interviews, those two months flew by. It was finally time to rank my programs. To be honest, I was a little nervous. I didn't have as many programs to choose from as I did when applying to PGY1 programs, and these programs had only one spot each. I created a list of pros and cons for each program. One program far outweighed the others. It was close to home, ranked the #1 children's hospital in the country, and had a history of matching PGY1 residents from my current program at the time. That was the program I ranked first. I just had to sit and wait patiently to find out if they felt the same way about me.

NOT MATCHING AND DESPAIR

The two weeks between program ranking and the match were the s l o w e s t two weeks of my life. It was all I could think about. Had I made the right decision with my ranking? I remember the morning of March 20, 2015 like it was yesterday. I was on my ambulatory care rotation sitting in on an antibiotic lecture. I watched the clock tick away on the wall. As text messages flooded my phone from my co-residents and friends also hearing about the match, I continued to refresh my email on my phone, wondering where my email was. During a class break, I finally saw the official email from the National Matching Service. I took a deep breath and opened it. I read the words "We regret to inform you..." and I couldn't breathe. Everything that I had been working toward for the past six years had come crashing down with those five ugly little words. How could I become a pediatric clinical pharmacist without completing a PGY2? My career was over before it even began. Well, not really, but that's what it felt like at the moment.

I knew I was destined to become a pediatric clinical pharmacist and had done everything in my power from the time I was in high school to achieve this goal. The rest of the day was rough. I had to go back to Tufts to facilitate a seminar for fourth-year pharmacy students. I had to face all of my co-residents and preceptors asking how the match went. I was the only one out of my residency class of five who didn't match in a PGY2 program. It was a day of celebration for everyone else so I did my best to be happy for them, but inside I was crushed. A few of my preceptors encouraged me to find out what pediatric PGY2 programs had not matched their spots. I wasn't feeling very motivated, but out of curiosity I decided to look. A few of the programs that didn't match were ones I had weeded out from my original list of programs. I thought that if I didn't feel they were right for me in the first place, why should I change my standards just because I didn't match? Feeling overwhelmed, I decided to take the weekend to self-reflect and decide whether or not I would try to scramble.

MOVING FORWARD

By Monday morning, my mind had been made up. I would not participate in the scramble and would start my search for a full-time clinical pharmacist position. I reached out to past preceptors and other contacts, and made connections with UConn alumni in the Boston area in hopes of finding a position. The managers at my hospital were aware of my fate. I expressed to one of the assistant directors my desire to stay at Tufts upon completion of my PGY1. He promised to keep me in mind as new positions opened up. We continued to have transparent conversations over the next few months regarding the availability at Tufts. Meanwhile, I applied and interviewed at the hospital where I completed my IPPE and one other. I was offered a second job interview at Charlton Memorial Hospital, a general medical and surgical hospital in Fall River, Massachusetts, and the place I got my start in hospital pharmacy. I loved it there, and knew I would feel right at home already knowing all of the pharmacy staff. However, it also meant giving up on my dream of becoming a pediatric clinical pharmacist, as that hospital did not provide care for pediatric patients. I talked to my assistant director again, and he offered me a per diem position working 40 hours a week in adult medicine. This offer was the deciding factor—I would stay at Tufts and hope that a pediatric clinical pharmacist position would eventually become available.

On the last day of my PGY1, I received a note from one of my preceptors complimenting me on the grace and resilience I displayed when dealing with the upset of not matching with a PGY2 program. I had never experienced adversity like that in my professional career, and it brought me much pride to see that others were impressed by the way I picked myself back up and moved forward with my career.

ACHIEVING MY GOAL

Fast forward three months later to September 2015, and a full-time clinical pharmacist position opened up in the pediatric satellite. I wrote a letter to the Tufts Medical Center pharmacy leadership team expressing my interest in the position and describing the skills and qualities I had to offer, and I was offered the position. I have been in this role for over two years now. Since accepting the position, I have had the opportunity to learn and grow as a pediatric pharmacist. I have rotated through the general pediatrics floor, pediatric intensive care unit, neonatal intensive care unit, and the pediatric bone marrow transplant unit. I am now the primary pharmacist for the general pediatrics floor, and I serve as the preceptor for that rotation for fourth-year pharmacy students and residents. I am also a member of the complex care committee and am precepting a resident on a project regarding the implementation of a pediatric antimicrobial stewardship program at the Floating Hospital for Children at Tufts Medical Center. Finally, I plan to sit for my board certification in pediatric pharmacotherapy this spring.

Not matching with a pediatric PGY2 residency program was definitely not the end of the world like it felt to me back on March 20, 2015. *After getting knocked down, I picked myself up, dusted myself off, and moved forward to achieve the career that I had dreamed of.* I refused to let this minor setback in my career get in the way of achieving my professional goals. Failure helped me to grow and develop resilience, which is an important skill to have in the workplace. I hope that my story resonates with many of you, and perhaps some of you can even relate to my experience. I would like to end my message to you with a quote by Elizabeth Edwards, as I feel it perfectly sums up my story of resilience in my early professional career. ***"She stood in the storm and when the wind did not blow her way, she adjusted her sails."***

Best wishes,

Brienne

Bethany Crouse
PharmD

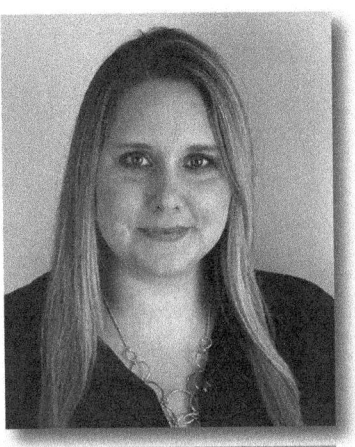

Walk in My Shoes

Bethany believes that a positive outlook is an essential trait of a successful pharmacist. Despite the stress and demands of residency training and clinical practice, she strives to maintain an enthusiastic perspective. Her upbeat demeanor and compassionate spirit allow her to connect to and gain the trust of her patients. Bethany is always accountable and does what is right, not what is easy. Her persistence has earned her the reputation as a reliable and knowledgeable colleague.

Bethany is currently a Critical Care Clinical Pharmacist at Vidant Medical Center, Greenville, North Carolina. She completed her accredited postgraduate year 2 (PGY2) critical care pharmacy residency at Vidant Medical Center and her accredited PGY1 pharmacy residency at Penn State Milton S. Hershey Medical Center, Hershey, Pennsylvania. Bethany received her PharmD degree from Lake Erie College of Osteopathic Medicine, School of Pharmacy, Pennsylvania and her BS in Animal Sciences at the Pennsylvania State University, University Park.

Bethany's advice is: **Whatever you choose to do with your future career, always be sure to make the most of today!**

Dear Pharmacy Colleague,

I've been in your shoes. I, too, have contemplated if residency training was the right choice

for me. *Will I be able to obtain a residency position? Do I have what it takes to be a successful resident?* I considered these questions carefully and evaluated all of my options before I made the decision to pursue residency training. Now, I want to give you the opportunity to walk in my shoes by sharing some of the experiences that helped to solidify my decision to apply for a pharmacy residency, as well as my residency experiences that confirmed I had made the right choice.

41

APRIL 2013

With the goal of challenging my clinical skills, I scheduled my first rotation as a pharmacy student at a large academic medical center. I have not had my first pharmacotherapy course yet, which means each clinical scenario I encounter is a new experience for me. Today, I will face a new level of clinical challenges rounding in the medical intensive care unit (ICU), and I will be asked many questions for which I will not know the answer. Today, I commit to approaching each patient with curiosity and enthusiasm.

Time passes quickly in the fast-paced ICU environment, where patients can decompensate with minimal warning. I remember one afternoon vividly: the life flight team arriving with a patient in cardiac arrest, actively receiving cardiopulmonary resuscitation. My mind races as I review Advanced Cardiac Life Support pathways in my head, attempting to comprehend everything happening simultaneously to this patient. Around me, countless healthcare professionals descend on the patient to provide care, working together as a team. I look to my preceptor, expecting to be told to stand aside and observe. Instead, he pulls me into the room and encourages me to be an active participant. I watch as he interacts with the team, calling out recommendations and anticipating therapy before it is even requested. My hands are shaking as he instructs me to properly prepare each medication. The physician at the bedside announces the patient is responding. It is an incredible feeling knowing that I was part of saving a life today.

Today was one of the most memorable experiences in my pharmacy career. The clinical knowledge and rapport that my preceptor had with his medical team was so impressive, demonstrating the importance of postgraduate training in becoming a confident clinician. This experience was an integral moment in my decision to pursue residency training. It was followed by many positive experiences in my clinical rotations, which also helped to solidify my decision. The application process was challenging, but the hardest work was still yet to come. I was blessed to match into a respected PGY1 residency program and couldn't wait to move on to the next stage in my career. My PGY1 residency year pushed me to the limits of my abilities and challenged me in both professional and personal ways. Amid a schedule filled with resident obligations, I had distinct experiences that had a profound impact on my development.

NOVEMBER 2015

Five months into my PGY1 residency, I am arguably in the most stressful part of the year, with numerous deadlines fast approaching. Today, I am rounding with the Trauma and Surgical Intensive Care team. Despite a solid foundation from my initial residency rotations, this month has already challenged me significantly as I manage one of the busiest ICU services in the hospital. Balancing patient care responsibilities with my resident obligations will be difficult, but I commit to stretching myself to overcome my limitations and grow in my independence as a clinician.

It's amazing how quickly time passes as a PGY1 resident. A schedule filled with patient care, presentations, student mentoring, and departmental meetings can easily consume my time. Sitting down one afternoon, I contemplate my future. In a few short weeks, I will be interviewing for PGY2 residency programs at the ASHP Midyear Clinical Meeting. In this moment, I feel many emotions—excitement about future opportunities, but also apprehension about the challenges ahead and my ability to meet the demands of a PGY2 program. Suddenly, my thoughts are interrupted by my pager announcing the impending arrival of a level I trauma victim, and I rush to the emergency department to join my team. They look to me to help devise the appropriate treatment strategy for this patient, confirming the value of my role as a member of the team. Walking back to my office, I consider how far I've come during my PGY1 residency. Today, I saw growth in my knowledge and confidence as a member of the medical team. I used my resources to find answers for a patient in critical need. My residency projects are still unfinished, and I haven't practiced my PGY2 interview questions yet, but I had a valuable impact on my patient. Today, I confirmed my desire to pursue a PGY2 in critical care.

MARCH 2016

Today is an important day. I will find out the results—I will find out the PGY2 residency match results, and I commit to remain positive. It's amazing how quickly time passed on Match Day. I hadn't slept well as I anxiously awaited the match results and I was sure the day would move slowly. Instead, I am called to the Heart and Vascular Intensive Care Unit for a rapidly decompensating patient. The perfusion team is called, and I have the opportunity to witness extracorporeal membrane oxygenation cannulation.

Today I matched into a PGY2 critical care residency program. I am overwhelmed with relief and yet anxious about the increased demands of a PGY2 program. Today, I thought my focus would be on Match Day. Instead, I was in awe as I witnessed the medical innovation of extracorporeal support and was humbled by the unique role of a pharmacist in evaluating pharmacotherapy in this patient population. Today, I am confident that a PGY2 critical care residency was the right decision for me.

———

The patient scenarios above were only a few of many exciting opportunities that I had during my PGY1 residency. I committed myself to making the most of every day as a resident, and my program supported me every step of the way. Transitioning to my PGY2 residency, I had countless experiences caring for critically ill patients and continued to strengthen my skills as a clinician. But I also found that my PGY2 residency challenged me outside of my clinical abilities. Successful pharmacists not only serve as vital medical team members, but also manage quality improvement projects; educate students, residents, and providers; and conduct valuable medical research. These skills can be some of the most difficult to master.

JANUARY 2017

Today I am not only a team member for the medical ICU service, but also the preceptor for my own pharmacy student. Over the past 6 months, my clinical skills have grown considerably. This month, I faced a new level of responsibility as I translated that knowledge to a learner.

Time passes quickly when you precept a student. Observing my student, I see many familiar traits from my own time as a student a few short years ago—excitement as she experiences patient scenarios previously only seen in a classroom, but also hesitation in her ability to make clinical recommendations. I have committed to help her get the most out of this rotation, the way my preceptors helped me. As we approach the end of bedside rounds, the unit is filled with alarms. We rush to the bedside to observe our patient struggling to breathe. I fight the urge to jump into action and instead pull my student into the room. As the team makes the decision to intubate the patient, I guide my student to consider her role in selecting appropriate medications for this procedure. I watch as she prepares the medications for the team, her hands shaking from the adrenaline. The procedure is performed successfully, and I watch as my student comprehends her role in caring for this patient.

Today I was able to step back and allow my student to apply her knowledge, make decisions, and execute them in a critical situation. I, too, expanded my skillset beyond clinical ability and moved closer to my goal to be a well-rounded clinical pharmacist.

One of the main goals of a residency program is to teach residents the skills they will need to be confident, independent practitioners. Looking back over my two years of residency training, I can see substantial growth in myself as a pharmacist. I was still anxious accepting my first pharmacist position after residency as I knew there would be a new level of responsibility without preceptor oversight. But I also knew I was well prepared to face the post-residency challenges ahead.

OCTOBER 2017

Today is October 16th—a day I had been anticipating for months. I will start a new service providing clinical pharmacy services to critically ill patients during evening hours. I collaborated with my colleagues to design this service to provide continuity of care for the sickest patients in the hospital, an unmet need in our institution. Physicians and nurses express their appreciation for having a clinical pharmacist at the bedside during evening hours, assisting with new ICU admissions, and facilitating complicated patient transfers from outside institutions. Today, I will be at the bedside when patients are decompensating and will assist my provider colleagues in making the best pharmacotherapy decisions during stressful situations. I will demonstrate to patients and their families that my institution is invested in providing the best patient care, no matter what time of day.

At the end of a long shift, I think about each of my interactions with both patients and providers. It amazes me how much I have changed in the few short years from when I stepped into that hospital for my first clinical rotation five years ago. I realize that I am now able to combine many skills gained through my residency training to improve care for my patients.

When I look back over the past several years, a pattern emerges: my true abilities emerge when I am faced with some of the steepest obstacles. *Residency training will inevitably present you with challenges; your success is determined by your response.* Each of my experiences that I shared with you required a conscious decision to make the most of a challenging situation, a decision that provided an opportunity for growth and helped to further shape my future.

I sincerely hope you have the opportunity to be a pharmacy resident and help save a life during cardiac arrest, witness medical innovation, or guide your own student to success as a pharmacist-in-training. Mostly, I hope you will have the opportunity to have a true impact on patients' lives. *Whatever you choose to do with your future career, always be sure to make the most of today!*

Best wishes,

Bethany

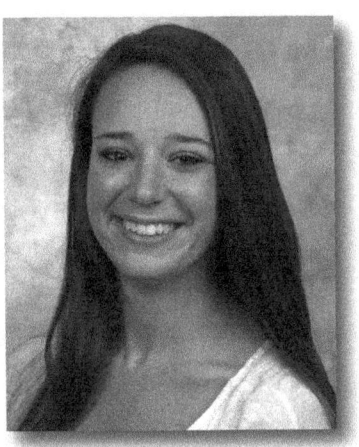

Jennifer Czerwinski
PharmD, MBA

Becoming the Shot Caller, Maximizing Feedback, and Learning from Mistakes

Jennifer is a driven, caring individual with an eye for detail and a heart of gold. Her MBA training allows her to carry herself in a mature manner, with a confident, yet approachable personality. Jennifer is a genuine and empathetic representative of her pharmacy department and the profession of pharmacy as a whole.

Jennifer is currently Staff Pharmacist at John Dempsey Hospital at UConn Health, Farmington, Connecticut. She completed her postgraduate year 1 (PGY1) pharmacy practice residency at John Dempsey Hospital. Jennifer received her BS and PharmD degrees from Western New England University College of Pharmacy, Springfield, Massachusetts and her MBA from Western New England University College of Business, Springfield, Massachusetts.

Jennifer's advice is: **Co-workers are the most important resource to gain your self-confidence to start calling the shots. Ask their opinions: what would they do and why? Understand the justification and reasoning from multiple perspectives, and you'll start to see yourself blossoming in your transition to a seasoned pharmacist.**

Dear Pharmacy Colleague,

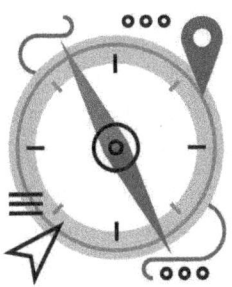

It's hard to believe that the time has finally come—that you finally sit at the crossroad between years of formal education and entering the workforce. If you're anything like me, you're probably excited, eager, and honestly a bit scared.

We've spent countless hours attending class, writing notes, memorizing the material, taking exams, and stressing. But despite the challenges and hard work, we made it! So why are we scared now to put it all into practice? As someone who is two and a half years into my career, I can tell you why—because patient lives are at stake. We know patient safety is the fundamental core of our profession, but somehow it is different now as we take our first steps as pharmacists and begin to call the shots. I want to let you know it's OK to be scared. As time passes, you will feel more comfortable and take on your role more naturally. Until then, you will have plenty of seasoned pharmacists to help you along the way. That's what residencies are for!

I may not have many years of experience, but what I do have to offer is a fresh perspective because I completed my PGY-1 residency less than two years ago. I can relate to what you will experience and feel because I was in your shoes what seems like just yesterday. Reflecting back on my residency year, there are so many things I learned clinically, professionally, and personally. You will be amazed at your progression after your residency year! In my humble opinion, the clinical and professional learning will come easy because most residency programs are structured to do just that. During your residency, you will have dedicated time to catch up on the most recent clinical guidelines, read and discuss journal articles with your preceptors and students, make evidence-based recommendations to your team, give presentations and complete a research project, as well as network with colleagues and attend professional meetings. It's the personal learning and growth that can sometimes fall by the wayside. I was extremely fortunate to have a program director, preceptors, and colleagues who didn't let me forget about my own personal needs and growth.

As you progress through your residency, keep these questions and thoughts in mind: When's the last time you visited home? Are you eating healthy or living off the quickest, cheapest thing you can find in the cafeteria? How are you balancing work, sleep, laundry, and fitness? When is the last time you spent time with your friends or significant other? Did you get your taxes done on time? When's the last time you called your grandma? I know these examples may seem like the least important things on your never ending to-do list, but don't underestimate them! It'll make a world of difference to have your personal life in-check. Plus, your grandma wants to hear from you and tell you how proud she is of you—and you need a cheerleader now more than ever!

There are a couple key things I'd like to share with you that I wish someone would've told me as I began my residency. I hope you find them helpful.

BECOMING THE SHOT CALLER

One of the biggest challenges I faced as a resident was taking on the full responsibility of being a pharmacist. I was nervous about the transition because I had always worked under someone's supervision. I was scared I wouldn't know the answer if asked a question, or that I would make the wrong judgment call when faced with a decision. This was very difficult for me in the beginning. I had worked so hard to get to this point in my career, but now I was hesitant to validate the safety and efficacy of patient orders, to put my signature of approval on a drug compounding record, or to check that an intravenous medication was appropriately prepared. I was scared to make a mistake and cause a patient harm.

Gaining the confidence and courage to finally "own" the responsibility of a pharmacist is something that will take time and experience. It will not be the same rate of progression in everyone, so don't be discouraged if your co-residents or former classmates appear to be more comfortable; chances are they feel just like you—you just can't see it because they don't show it! Use your resources to help you become more confident in yourself and in your work. This is not limited to books, online databases, clinical guidelines, or journal articles but rather trusted colleagues and mentors. Pharmacists, young and old, all felt like you do when they started their careers.

I found that my co-workers were the most important resource in gaining my own self-confidence to start calling the shots. Ask their opinions: what would they do and why? Understand the justification and reasoning from multiple perspectives, and you'll start to see yourself blossoming in your transition.

As a relatively new pharmacist, there are still plenty of times and situations in which I find myself tasked with calling the shots—the one with the final say. This often occurs when management and administration are not present (evenings, overnights, weekends, holidays), but can also occur while you are managing technicians, precepting students, leading a project, or starting a new role or position. The skills learned and developed during this crucial time will prepare you for bigger challenges in the future, so embrace them!

MAXIMIZING FEEDBACK

During your residency year, you'll be receiving feedback in a myriad of ways including formal evaluations from your preceptors and program director, from attendees of the profession at meetings or conferences in which you present, and from informal day-to-day conversations with your co-workers. Of course, the most challenging part of receiving feedback is hearing the areas for improvement. As difficult as it may be, I urge you to gracefully accept these truths and use them to improve your skillset. It does neither you nor the person giving the feedback any good to blanket the evaluation with a "Great job!" and send you on your way. That would be a disservice to your future growth.

We've all heard of the *feedback sandwich* which contains positive comments, areas of improvement, and then finished with more positive comments. Personally I think this is a great feedback tool because it allows me to identify where I can improve without crushing my self-confidence along the way. But I never considered seeking feedback on my own, without the prompting of a midway or final evaluation. Ask your preceptors after your first week (and weekly thereafter) what you have done well and what they would like to see you work on. I think we often interpret feedback as formalized evaluations, but it can be as simple as asking pharmacists around you how they think you are performing. The advantage is that you know exactly where you stand every time you ask for feedback, not once the learning experience has ended.

Feedback should also be mutual when appropriate. Your residency program has many more years to continue educating the future members of our profession, and as preceptors, we want to make sure we're doing a good job, too! Again, either through formalized evaluations of your preceptors or just daily discussions let them know what it is you find helpful. What aspects of their precepting do you enjoy? What are some ways they could improve to create a better learning experience for future residents and students? You may even find yourself emulating these attributes when you have students or residents of your own. One simple thing that made an immense impact on my residency year was "Feedback Fridays" in which I would join my co-resident, program director, clinical coordinator, and manager for lunch every Friday. Our dialogue constantly evolved as we progressed through the year, starting with how our orientation and training were going all the way through manuscript writing and post-residency career pursuits. We all found this to be a powerful tool to ensure open communication and mutual feedback.

LEARNING FROM MISTAKES

Let's get one thing straight: everyone makes mistakes. And, yes, that includes me, you, and every other pharmacist; even everyone who graduated with a 4.0 GPA. I don't need to tell you that the technology introduced into our profession has made a tremendous impact on patient safety and undoubtedly will continue to do so. But it's not foolproof, and it's not perfect. Unfortunately, mistakes do still happen.

Two of the most important lessons I learned in making mistakes of my own are to be transparent and be a patient advocate. Transparency is everything when it comes to a mistake. What was the error? Did it reach the patient? What factors contributed to the error being made? These are just a few of the surface level questions that should come to mind when a mistake, yours or someone else's, is discovered. I had wonderful medication safety preceptors who always emphasized that an error should never be blamed on an individual's knowledge or competence, but rather the multitude of factors that came together to allow the error to occur. It is a vital perspective to have to prevent the error from happening again and where the patient advocacy piece comes in. Once the contributing factors of the error are identified, how will you ensure that they are addressed and/or fixed? I will never forget when I inadvertently verified an intravenous antibiotic order with an "as needed" status, never prompting the nurse to administer the dose. The event was brought to the team and the patient's attention, and it was discovered that the computerized order entry system had been erroneously built to set this medication "as needed" anytime it was ordered. In other words, this was not an isolated event due to my lack of knowledge, but an error that would occur every time if not addressed by the primary factors contributing to the error. I worked with our information technology (IT) department closely until I had full certainty and validation that the system was corrected. So I urge you, always be careful and cautious, but when a mistake occurs, remain transparent and focus on being an advocate for your patient and the patients to come.

Like other aspects of your life, you need to maintain happy and healthy relationships within the profession. I'm sure you've already seen what a small world pharmacy really is! Be sure to establish good relationships with the people you work with, from the technicians and students all the way to the pharmacy director. These positive connections will lead to better teamwork, a happier career, and even professional opportunities in the future. After all, that's how I was offered the chance to write you this letter!

Wishing you the best of luck in your endeavors,

Jennifer

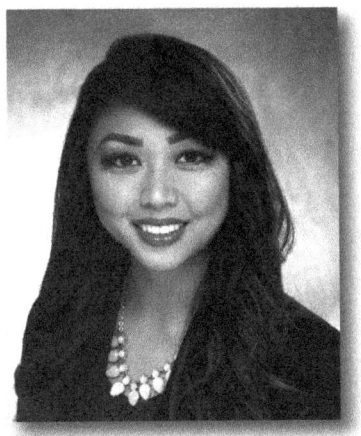

Jessica M. Dizon
PharmD, MHA, BCPS

The Rite of Rejection—Persistence, Resilience, and Patience Prevail

Jessica traces her career direction to her mother who aspired to be a pharmacist but circumstances prohibited. Jessica experienced a string of setbacks in her journey through college, pharmacy school, and residency selection. However, in spite of these obstacles, she demonstrated her tenacity to achieve her goals and have a successful career.

Jessica is currently an Ambulatory Clinical Coordinator at CareOregon in Portland, Oregon, one of Oregon's managed care organizations serving Medicaid and Medicare populations. Jessica completed a postgraduate year 1 (PGY1) pharmacy and PGY2 health-system pharmacy administration (HSPA)/MHA residency at the University of Iowa Hospitals and Clinics and the University of Iowa College of Public Health. She received her PharmD from the University of New England in Portland, Maine and her BS in Biology from the University of California, Santa Cruz (UCSC).

Jessica's advice is: ***Despite obstacles and rejections in your planned career path, persistence in meeting your goals and the development of leadership skills will ultimately allow you to have a successful career.***

Dear Pharmacy Colleague,

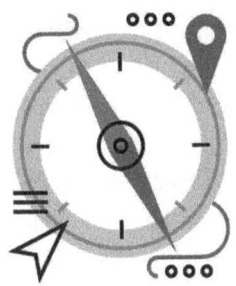

Rejection is oftentimes synonymous with failure—rejection from your choice of colleges, pharmacy schools, or not matching into a residency program or fellowship. These scenarios are all too familiar for me. The lessons that I learned and the relationships I formed have stemmed from episodes of rejection and failure. Rejections and failures are an inevitable component of life, but they don't define you as a person. What defines you—what shapes you into the person you are destined to be—are the actions and steps you have taken in the face of those obstacles. During those difficult times, it's tough to see the light at the end of the tunnel. You start to reflect, dissect, and analyze every decision and second-guess your life choices. From direct experience, I can say, "Everything will be okay." I faced rejection at many critical points in my adult life, but you must pick yourself up and make the decision to stay the course, find a new route, or pivot into unchartered territory. Life happens, things change, and there are no guarantees. Despite disappointments, we must learn to adapt in order to be successful.

My education and career journey has not been a straight path from Point A to Point B. My path to pharmacy began before I was born. As a first-generation Filipino-American, there is often an unspoken parental pressure to succeed. For many of us, our parents have preconceived notions about what defines success, and the general school of thought is that it can only be achieved through higher education to become doctors and lawyers. Our parents have sacrificed their own opportunities to give their children the chance to have better, more successful lives. My mother aspired to become a pharmacist, but when she moved to the United States from the Philippines, she had to help support her family. At 18 years old, she and my grandfather went to work while my grandmother stayed at home to care for their five other children. My mother put her dreams on hold; although she never became a pharmacist, she worked at different pharmaceutical companies as a quality assurance supervisor, and continually pitched the idea of me becoming a pharmacist. However, growing up, I wasn't sure that I wanted to become a pharmacist. All I knew is that I wanted to help people, and I could reach them through healthcare.

The first obstacle I faced in my journey came during my senior year of high school—I had applied to seven colleges and received six rejection letters. But then, finally, in April I received an email from the University of California, Santa Cruz. I had been accepted and was to begin my journey in the fall. Before I knew it, I had my Bachelor's degree in Biology and no clue what I was going to do next.

EXPLORING NEW PATHS AND FACING REJECTION HEAD-ON

When I initially left for college, I promised myself I would never move back home; yet, there I was—back in Southern California and completely lost. It wasn't long before the pharmacy career "seeds," which my mother planted over many years, took hold. I decided to test the waters and took a job as a pharmacy technician in a long-term care pharmacy. The pharmacists I worked with demonstrated the amazing care they provide for patients, and I realized that this was the career for me. It took another two years before I was accepted to the University of New England, a new pharmacy school on the other side of the country in Portland, Maine. Going to a newly established pharmacy school had its advantages as well as its disadvantages. The advantages included leadership opportunities, expansion of national student organizations on our campus, and the ability to shape the course of our program through executive board meetings. The disadvantages in new schools often include a lack of postgraduate residency education opportunities and few alumni for guidance, an obstacle that was not made clear to me until I decided to pursue a health-system pharmacy administration residency (HSPA) in my fourth year.

Many of the established HSPA programs are located in the Midwest. Because I was from the West Coast, and had studied on the East Coast, I had zero connections in pharmacy administration. Little did I know as a student pharmacist that networking can change the course of one's career. Building your network can help make connections with an array of individuals with disparate backgrounds and careers similar to the ones you wish to pursue. These seemingly insignificant encounters can manifest into mentorships and/or friendships that can help you navigate your career. The value of networking had not crossed my mind until it was too late. Match Day came, and my mind went blank after I read the first few words, "We regret to inform you...." Again, I was faced with rejection, but instead of moping, I sat down and developed my game plan. In my search, I came across the University of Iowa Hospitals and Clinics (UIHC). I had never considered moving to Iowa, and during my first search, the program was not even on my radar. The week of the Residency Scramble was chaotic and frustrating but altogether enlightening. In that short week, I learned a lot about resilience, persistence, and patience. The following Monday, I received a call from my would-be mentor and residency program director, Mike Brownlee, the Chief Pharmacy Officer at UIHC, offering me a position as one of the PGY1/PGY2 health-system pharmacy administration residents—I gladly accepted.

The day that I moved to Iowa was the first time I had visited the state, and orientation day was the first time I had ever stepped into the hospital. There, I would dedicate two years to strengthening my clinical knowledge and developing my leadership skills through projects and completion of my PGY1/PGY2 HSPA residency and Masters of Health Administration. The life skills I had gained from overcoming different obstacles would help prepare me for the challenges residency would bring. As time went on, I started to narrow my focus to clinical management because I had always enjoyed the clinical aspects of being a pharmacist, but I wanted to effect change at a higher level. After my first year, I sat for the Board Certification Exam in Pharmacotherapy (BCPS) because I wanted to prove to myself that I had a strong clinical foundation and I wanted to add validity to my training. During my second year, I focused on developing my analytical aptitude, project management skills, and those softer skills that would help me to be an effective communicator and leader. Residency pushed me to the limits both physically and mentally with countless hours dedicated to class assignments and intensive department projects such the opening of a brand-new Children's Hospital. The timing of these major projects coincided with planning the next stage of my life: finding a career position.

SEARCHING FOR A CAREER POSITION

Pursuing my new career brought an additional layer of stress into my life. I knew I wanted to find a position that would play into my strengths; I knew that I wanted a job in clinical management. As the job search began, the market for clinical managers was smaller than I had anticipated. Luckily, my residency training gave me the skills to think strategically, and I adjusted my search to positions that had opportunities interfacing with clinical management. I had applied for over 10 positions, heard back from five, interviewed for three, and was offered one. Even though I had an offer on the table, I still had one position pending. I found a position at CareOregon, a managed care organization in Portland; I had never worked in managed care before and knew little about the business model, but it met my criteria for opportunities that interfaced with clinical management. I knew I would work with patients as well as have the ability to develop and participate in new and innovative projects. CareOregon offered me the opportunity to see an avenue of pharmacy that was foreign to me but would allow flexibility in forging a new path. *This was a pivotal point in my life—either I had to accept the offer on the table or take a risk on a potential position in an unfamiliar setting.* In the end, I decided to take the risk and move forward with the interview process at CareOregon. All of my "eggs" were in the CareOregon basket; if they decided to move forward with another candidate, I'd be back to square one.

I accepted a position at CareOregon in May and began my new journey at the end of July. My position would be serving as the transitions pharmacist for two rural coordinated care organizations (CCOs) in Oregon. Transitions of care is new to these rural CCOs, and I am able to use my experience working within a large health system to help manage the workflow for patients transitioning post-discharge. In my current role, I work with a multidisciplinary group across different healthcare systems to improve transitions of care that will have a positive impact on patient outcomes. CareOregon serves the Medicaid and Medicare population with patients who have chronic, severe illnesses as well as challenging social determinants that require additional resources. My work is a hybrid of ambulatory care clinical coordination and meeting the health plan's needs. For the health plan side of business, we analyze our patient's utilization (medications, emergency department visits, inpatient stays, etc.) and develop strategies to decrease unnecessary utilization and improve patient outcomes.

Our work is data-driven, and my residency training helped me approach my work in a logical, methodical way that can aid process improvement to streamline the work. Even though the area of managed care pharmacy was new to me, residency training prepared me to be successful by providing skills in data analytics, effective communication, and process improvement strategies as well as a creating a strong clinical foundation. My current position allows me to work in a dynamic environment that is open to new ideas, strives for innovation, and advocates for our patients. I never thought I would end up in the position I have now, but it has all the components I want and need to grow in my career.

My life is drastically different than what I imagined back in high school, college, pharmacy school, and even at the start of residency, just a mere two years ago. The steps I took after the rejections I encountered brought me to different areas of the country, gave me the opportunity to grow my pharmacy network, brought me to a residency program that ended up being a perfect match, and led me to a position and, ultimately, a career I love. Along the way I have formed invaluable friendships, and I sit here today with no regrets.

Times of rejection may seem like the end of the world, but if you keep an open mind, stay resilient, and keep a positive outlook, you may find yourself in a new and exciting adventure. Sometimes it takes a leap of faith, but in the end you will get to where you need to go.

Wishing you success,

Jessica

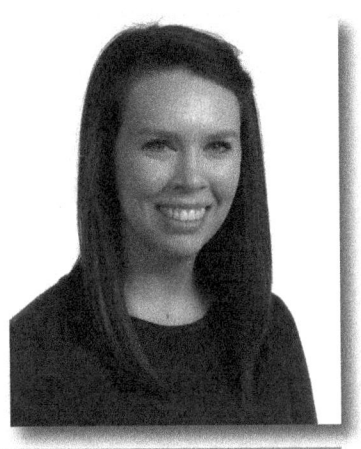

Erin Graham
PharmD

Navigating the Decision Tree to Find Your Ideal Practice Setting

Erin reflects on her own experiences in choosing a profession, type of pharmacy practice, residency, and practice setting as she develops her career. She provides guidance on navigating your own path to a happy and rewarding career.

Erin is a Project Specialist Pharmacist at Balls Food Stores Pharmacies in Kansas City, Kansas and Missouri. She received her PharmD degree from the University of Kansas School of Pharmacy and completed a postgraduate year 1 (PGY1) residency in community pharmacy at the University of Kansas School of Pharmacy and Balls Food Stores, in Kansas City, Kansas.

Erin's advice is: *Keep your eyes wide open, and give honest consideration to all career opportunities along the way. Choose to pursue those opportunities that bring you the most joy for a happy and satisfying career.*

Dear Pharmacy Colleague,

CHOOSING PHARMACY

I assume your goal is to become an excellent pharmacist with a great career. You are

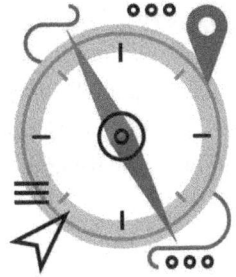

in a fun, challenging, exciting, and somewhat scary spot. As someone who made it through the season of life that is pharmacy school, residency, and landing that first post-residency job, I hope to share my experiences that you may find useful. I do not come from a pharmacy or even healthcare family. I had a difficult time deciding what career direction to pursue. Thankfully, my parents had heard a pharmacy career was a rewarding one so, at their encouragement I shadowed and interviewed pharmacists to get a first-hand look. After that limited exposure, I was intrigued and found myself a job at a compounding pharmacy where I discovered pharmacy was a great fit for me. As a career, it provided the best job attributes rolled into one—serving people, building meaningful relationships with patients, making positive changes in patients' health, and utilizing my math and science-loving brain to solve problems and challenges every day. I can't express the relief I felt after deciding to pursue pharmacy. I thought all the hard decisions were over, and I had finally picked my career path. *What else was left to choose?*

CHOOSING A PRACTICE TYPE

I had placed rose-colored glasses squarely over my eyes. I was wrong to think all my career decisions were finished and behind me. It's true, as a pharmacist, I get to build positive patient relationships and utilize my "science" brain to help patients improve their health in many ways. But those glasses were rosier than ever as I thought my hardest career decision was deciding to become a pharmacist. After my first day of pharmacy school, I realized the real decision making and soul searching had yet to begin. The hardest decision I would wrestle with was choosing the *setting or type of practice* I would pursue. I had done extensive research before selecting pharmacy as a profession, but all my research didn't prepare me for the overwhelming number of practice options following graduation. As I became involved in various pharmacy organizations, I met many successful, accomplished pharmacists making concrete contributions to the profession and their patients. Exposure to these pharmacists and learning about their career paths helped me to define the *type* of pharmacist I wanted to be. I wanted to become the *type* of pharmacist who built strong, positive patient relationships, operated on the front lines (primary care), found creative solutions to tough problems, endeavored to become a leader, and implemented successful, financially sustainable patient care programs.

The problem arrived when I found this *type* or those characteristics among pharmacists in every aspect of the pharmacy profession. I met such role models at national conferences including ASHP and the American Pharmacists Association. I met them in my own school in networking sessions that I helped to orchestrate with the Student Society of Health-System Pharmacy and in volunteering to precept health fairs for the American Pharmacists Association Academy of Student Pharmacists. My biggest dilemma was the realization that the type of pharmacist I strived to be was not limited to an individual field of pharmacy practice. Thus, the real question remained: *Where* would I enjoy striving to be that type of pharmacist—hospital, managed care organization, ambulatory care clinic, compounding pharmacy, community pharmacy, or perhaps a drug information center?

CHOOSING A PRACTICE SETTING AND RESIDENCY PROGRAM

Choosing the environment of practice became the overwhelming question. I didn't know where to start so I dabbled in everything. During school you could find me in at least one committee meeting for just about every club offered. I worked as a student pharmacist in both a VA hospital and an independently owned community pharmacy. Throughout my organizational involvement and job experiences, it became apparent a residency program following graduation was the next critical step. This decision could propel me toward becoming the pharmacist I strived to be. However, I felt residency programs for my specific interests were not plentiful. I really enjoyed practice in a community pharmacy, and I was most happy on advanced pharmacy practice experience (APPE) rotations when a patient learned my name and asked for me the next time they visited. The long-term relationships you are able to build in the community setting, with patients returning month after month, brings me the most joy in my job today. I cherish this relationship. However, the majority of pharmacy residency programs are set in a health-system environment. The chatter among my respected classmates involved which health-system residency program they were applying to. I felt like the odd ball out. I didn't know how to reconcile my career aspirations with the pharmacy setting that brought me the most joy.

FINDING MENTORS AND MAKING A DECISION

This is where I hope to remind you of a well-known phrase, "You don't know what you don't know." As a student I had a limited understanding of the challenges facing the pharmacy profession, the climate of the healthcare system, and the changing demands placed on pharmacy practice. It wasn't the classroom that helped me unravel my uncertainty in choice of practice site, it was my experience at national conferences both health system and community focused. My didactic education was excellent in preparing me for the practice of pharmacy as a clinician. My organizational involvement was what prepared me for the profession of pharmacy. Sitting at meetings and listening to experienced pharmacists discuss new initiatives helped me understand the opportunities and types of jobs available. It developed my understanding of our profession's needs and the changing needs of our patients. It facilitated my introduction to positive mentors who provided guidance and advice as I tried to navigate my career choices. People who have weathered the storm before you make for excellent guides. It is these mentors I gained along the way who opened the door for me to see the development of advanced pharmacy practices in community pharmacies. In fact, it was my involvement in professional organizations that introduced me to the University of Kansas and Balls Food Stores community residency program where I matched and went on to be hired following completion of my residency. In the end, all of my decision points along the way were, indeed, preparing me to make the appropriate choices for me.

DEVELOPING MY REWARDING PRACTICE

After many conferences and meetings listening to accomplished pharmacists speak, I started to realize community pharmacy had become the new frontier. There I found a *new kind of pharmacist* to take on the different challenges in this practice setting. Although much of pharmacy practice grew from the iconic neighborhood drug store, community pharmacy is being reinvented as a place of direct patient care and readily accessible clinical services. Community-based pharmacy practice exists today in a healthcare environment drastically different from that of the recent past. The business model is changing, the needs of our patients are changing, and the healthcare environment itself is demanding more of community-based pharmacy care.

I now enjoy the challenge of developing into an innovative, patient-centered, business savvy and creative clinician in community practice. The key word here is *enjoy*! Community pharmacy practice brings me joy, which gives me the stamina to continue toward my lofty goals of making a positive impact on the profession. My current position allows me to work the front lines at the pharmacy counter and develop positive patient relationships. Yes, I know my patients by name, and they know my name as their pharmacist. I am also afforded the time and opportunity to develop programs for our community-based grocery store pharmacy department. Currently, I am implementing initiatives to provide patients their medications in adherence packages, providing Medicare Part D open enrollment counseling, teaching diabetes education classes, precepting pharmacy students, providing medication therapy management services, and developing direct patient care clinical activities for our current resident. I think all of these are stepping stones in my goal to be that type of pharmacist I envisioned.

My day at work is fun, enjoyable, and rewarding for reasons such as the same couple who attend my diabetes education classes also ask for my advice on their Medicare Part D plan enrollment and recommendations on their vaccination profile. I get to pair that unique patient–pharmacist relationship with the fun and exciting expansion of clinical services. I can't claim to have crossed the finish line in becoming that type of pharmacist I desire. I'm really just getting started. But I can say I've found the environment and practice setting that brings me the joy and satisfaction to propel me toward that goal. Although I find the excitement of innovation and creativity in the community-based practice setting, the same energy is buzzing in every other *type* of pharmacy practice setting.

Find the place in pharmacy that makes you happy, wherever that may be. Personally, that "happy place" for me is found inside your neighborhood drug store down the street. My hope is that you take from this letter a few nuggets to help you on your journey:

- The *type* of pharmacist you become is not limited to or defined by your practice setting.

- Select your practice setting based on what brings you joy and happiness!

- Set your sights high. Find your *type* of pharmacist and navigate to become that pharmacist.

- You don't know what you don't know. Learn about your profession, not just the practice. Pharmacy school is the best place to learn about the practice of pharmacy. Involvement in the profession and organizations is the best place to learn about the profession of pharmacy.

I wish you all the best!

Erin

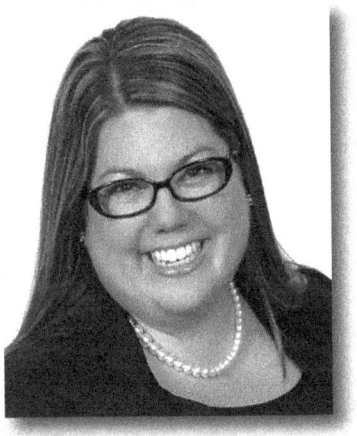

Brigid K. Groves
PharmD, MS

Knock, Knock! Who's There? Unexpected Career Opportunities

Brigid developed a passion for administration and leadership in community pharmacy practice. She wanted to pursue a residency and graduate education in this area, but there were no options. But she became an inaugural resident–graduate student in the first national program established to meet her needs. She shares anxieties, opportunities, and successes as a pioneer in this program as well as her journey in developing her own career.

Brigid is currently Pharmacy Practice Coordinator for The Kroger Co., Columbus Division, Assistant Professor and Residency Program Director, The Ohio State University College of Pharmacy, Columbus, Ohio. She completed her postgraduate year 1 (PGY1) community pharmacy and PGY2 community pharmacy administration/MS residencies and graduate degree at The Ohio State University College of Pharmacy in Columbus. She also holds her PharmD degree from The Ohio State University College of Pharmacy and a BS in Chemistry from John Carroll University in Cleveland, Ohio.

Brigid's advice is: *Share your goals with others; embrace and own the unknown; listen for the knock on the door for opportunities; always put the patient first; and most importantly, be upfront when your capacity isn't what it usually is.*

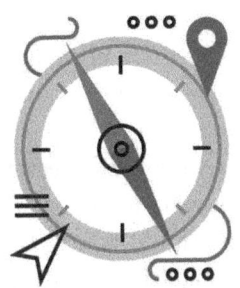

Dear Pharmacy Colleague,

"Time of death: 9:32 am." The words came so harshly to my ears, even though the nurse practitioner was trying to be caring and respectful. My mom passed away on December 30, 2016 from complications associated with a rare form of cancer known as epithelioid angiomyolipoma. It was as if the past two years of her battle collided into one moment and then sucked all of the air from my lungs. As my dad, two brothers, and my husband stood around my mom in intensive care, we realized we were blessed to be with her as she left this earthly body, but so unfortunate to have lost our rock at the tender age of 63. The next few weeks into months were a blur of condolences, packing up my parent's house, and getting finances in order.

Be upfront when your capacity isn't what it usually is. I had many well-meaning friends and colleagues tell me to "stay strong." When you lose someone so close to you, it is nearly impossible to stay strong. In my opinion, don't stay strong when you physically or mentally cannot. Take the time you need to heal from a difficult situation. However, it is important to let your friends, family, colleagues, and supervisor know that you are doing your best but cannot function at full capacity. My supervisor and work colleagues were incredibly supportive and understanding of my diminished capacity. My mother's death has taught me many lessons; in terms of my pharmacy career, I realized that I could still be successful in the long term, even if I could only ensure that the minimum aspects of my job were completed, while allowing others to take on the more thought-intensive tasks in the short term.

You are probably wondering by now what I actually do and what gives me the credibility to be writing a letter guiding your pharmacy residency selection and early career decision process. Don't fret; I'm getting there!

First, I'd like to share some tips that helped me develop and navigate my career and hopefully will help as you start the next steps of your career:

- Share with others your goals and passions.

- Embrace and own the unknown, design the process or solution, and celebrate the outcomes.

- Listen for the knock at the door and open it.

- Always put the patient first.

- Be upfront when your capacity isn't what it usually is.

When I entered pharmacy school, I fully intended to return to pharmaceutical industry where I had started as a quality control chemist. However, I had an early rotation experience at a traditional community pharmacy that made me realize how much I loved working directly with patients. I saw the impact that a pharmacist could have on these patients and wanted to provide this same level of patient care; thus, my focus changed to community pharmacy practice. While in pharmacy school, I became very involved in student organizations and had an opportunity to plan a regional meeting for student pharmacists. It was then I developed my passion for administration and leadership. I became aware of health-system pharmacy administration (HSPA) residency programs during my third year of pharmacy school and quickly realized this was an ideal way for me to develop a leadership and administration skillset specific for pharmacy practice. However, existing programs were all in hospital or health-system environments, not in community practice. I decided to focus on programs that had a stronger ambulatory care and outpatient pharmacy experience associated with them.

Share with others your goals and passions. As an advanced pharmacy practice experience (APPE) student, I continually shared my career goal of community phar-macy administration and my plan to pursue such a residency with my preceptors. One preceptor challenged my plan of obtaining a traditional HSPA residency because it was obvious my passion was in the community setting. He asked if I was familiar with a new program that was "HSPA-like," but it was a PGY1/PGY2 program in community pharmacy administration and leadership. The preceptor said they were searching for the ideal first candidate. This revelation piqued my interest, and my preceptor facil-itated a meeting with then program director, Marialice Bennett. I ended up applying and was subsequently selected as the first resident in this innovative program. Had I not continually shared my career goal and passion for community practice, I can't be sure that I would have learned about this residency until it was too late. It is important to share your goals and passions because you never know how someone's knowledge and network can help facilitate new directions.

Although I was extremely excited and honored to be the first resident in this program, I was also a bit hesitant. Because it had just begun, the program was unac-credited, the learning experiences and associated activities were unwritten, and the job market for a graduate of this program was unknown. Prior to starting this program, I would have said that I didn't like change or the unknown. However, experiences in an unknown area helped me develop a passion for starting something new and seeing it through to fruition. Being a pioneer can be exciting.

Embrace and own the unknown. I was lucky to have seasoned pharmacy practi-tioners leading me in this process. As a team, we composed standards, designed activ-ities, and wrote learning experiences. It was a rewarding experience to be in the initial creation and development of the residency program, and then complete them during my day-to-day in residency. Upon finishing the program, the program director applied for accreditation, and I had the opportunity to participate in the preparation for and day-of activities for the on-site accreditation visit. Talk about a nerve-wracking inter-view—imagine you are now a former resident explaining your experiences, activities, and projects to a team of well-established and respected pharmacists who are experts in residency training. We were ecstatic to learn that the Commission on Credentialing accredited the PGY1/PGY2/MS in community pharmacy administration and leader-ship program for the full six years! I had decided to embrace and own the unknown, worked with a team to design the process, and celebrated our success with accredita-tion and continuation of the program.

Listen for a knock on the door. Upon graduation, one of my mentors from residency offered me a clinical coordinator position at Kroger Pharmacy in Columbus, Ohio, where I completed my residency. I accepted this offer because it aligned with my career goal of working in community practice and helping patients through the pharmacists I taught, coached, and trained. I started my career focusing on the biometric screening program, intern program, and transitions of care services. I was just getting comfortable in my role and reflecting on where I wanted my career to grow, when there was a knock on the door.

Marialice was retiring and was curious if I was interested in serving as residency program director (RPD) for the PGY1/PGY2 program. I was floored that she thought to consider me for this role. I reflected on her offer; the goal of becoming an RPD was one I had considered, but didn't think it would be this early in my career. I also talked to my other mentors before I made the decision to accept the offer with her guidance. For me, I answered the knock because I wanted to ensure the program's continuation and growth. You never know when someone will knock on the door. My advice is to respond to the knock, evaluate its alignment with your goals and passions, and then decide on your answer.

Focus on the whole patient. In my career, my focus is on the whole patient, and I encourage my pharmacists to have that same focus. We did not go to pharmacy school or into community practice to simply "count by 5s." We went to provide patient care. I believe that my community-based pharmacist practitioners are essential healthcare providers in their neighborhoods. When working with my pharmacy teams, I step into workflow to build rapport and trust with the team and demonstrate patient-first behaviors. As a leader, it is essential that your team trusts you so that when you assign tasks, they know you won't require them to do more than you could do yourself. It is important to balance the administrative side of my practice with the priority of patient care and clinical activities. As you start making choices about your career path, determine the ideal balance for you. However, recognize that no matter what you do, the priority and focus is the patient.

To conclude, you never know what life has in store for you and your career. You may have plans to go one way, but then life happens and, suddenly, your path changes. It is important to make sure you *tell others about your goals and passions, embrace and own the unknown, open the door when there is a knock, and keep patients first. Finally, ensure that you share with others when your capacity is not what it usually is due to a situation beyond your control.* Both tragedy and personal loss can occur, and yet you learn to recover. Opportunities present themselves unexpectedly as you navigate your career.

Through the advice presented, you will be prepared. Residency truly opened many doors for me and helped me develop a professional network that I tap into regularly as I continue in my career. I wish you the best of luck in your residency, initial career search, and journey!

Take care,

Brigid

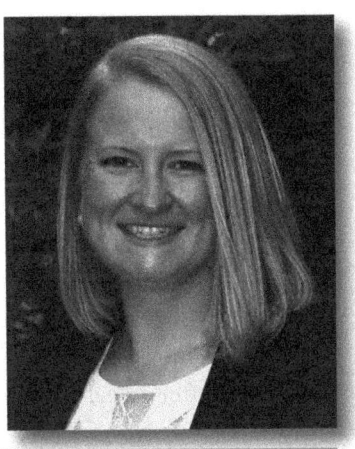

Chelsea Gustafson
PharmD, BCOP

Selecting the Right Residencies for a Dual Pharmacist Couple and Creating the Learning Experiences You Want

Chelsea is creative, adaptable, compassionate, determined, and passionate about our profession. She outlines how she selected pharmacy, health-system practice, and residency training. As a little "l" leader, she has worked to start and lead a new service for ambulatory oncology patients.

Chelsea is currently an Outpatient Oncology Clinical Pharmacist at Northwestern Medicine–Downtown Campus, Chicago, Illinois. She completed an accredited postgraduate year 1 (PGY1) pharmacy practice residency and an accredited PGY2 hematology/oncology pharmacy residency at Northwestern Memorial Hospital, having received her PharmD from Purdue University, College of Pharmacy, West Lafayette, Indiana.

Chelsea's advice is: **Love what you do, immerse yourself in what you are learning, and through your experiences, decide who you want to become as a pharmacist.**

Dear Pharmacy Colleague,

When I was in pharmacy school, I thought of the stereotypical pharmacist as a type A person who knew exactly where (s)he would be and what (s)he would be doing in 10 years, and I also knew that description did not fit me. I think

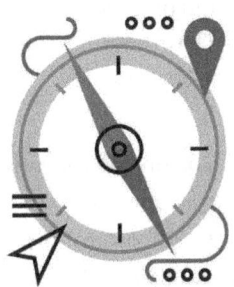

that there are far more pharmacists out there like me who do not know exactly what they want to do far in advance, and sometimes not even until they are already doing it, but fall in love with their career and choices as they make them. My story is one of loving what I do, immersing myself in what I am learning, and allowing myself to decide who I wanted to become as a pharmacist through my experiences.

I am the first person in my family to become a pharmacist or work in healthcare. When I was in high school, my best friend Kristyn knew exactly what she wanted to do—be a pharmacist. I had a much foggier view of my future self, but her desire and clarity about her decision made me want to find out why she wanted it so badly, so I looked into it. I shadowed a community pharmacist and saw his compassion for his patients and how his patients loved their pharmacist. After seeing that relationship, I became interested in pharmacy, too. I looked into college programs and decided to go to Purdue. I wanted a career helping others, but I did not know until I submitted my application and chose pre-pharmacy if that would be as a pharmacist or a math teacher. After 2 years of pre-pharmacy courses, I knew what I wanted and applied to Purdue's pharmacy school.

I honestly did not know anything about health-system pharmacy until I heard some of my professors talk about it. Residency was discussed all the time, but I hadn't really thought about it until I went to Kenya for two months for an advanced pharmacy practice experience (APPE) rotation and practiced in a hospital there. It was my first rotation, and I learned a lot about myself and who I was as a pharmacist. I gained a deeper understanding of the impact that a pharmacist could have by advocating for their patients and learned that I could do the same. After returning to the states, I decided to pursue residency.

I loved the environment that residency-trained pharmacists, preceptors, and residency-bound students created at ASHP's Midyear Clinical Meeting. I applied and interviewed with several PGY1 programs. I still remember walking out of the interview at Northwestern, thinking "this is it." I could feel the passion that everyone at Northwestern had for their patients and for being a pharmacist. Northwestern was where I wanted to be and where I felt like I belonged.

I met my husband, Joe, at Purdue in pharmacy school. He is my favorite person and biggest supporter. He is also, as you probably figured out, a pharmacist. Because we were in the same field, it was often easier for us to understand what the other was going through, but it also made the search for PGY1 and PGY2 quite a bit more complicated. For PGY1, we decided that we would focus on two cities, Chicago and Indianapolis, and from there, we would work with whatever hand was dealt to us. There was a chance we would be in two different cities, but we accepted that and decided not to do the couples match so that we could do what we each thought was best for our careers. Residency was only a year, and we knew that our relationship could withstand distance as we both advanced our careers in a way that only residency could.

I matched with Northwestern for PGY1 and was so excited! Fortunately, Joe also matched in Chicago so we moved there together. I started training and soon it was time to pick my rotations. We had a fantasy football-like draft to pick our rotations, which was great because it meant that I had a say in what my year would look like. Late in my last year of school, I had an APPE rotation in pediatric hematology and stem cell transplant that I absolutely loved. However, I honestly had no idea whether I loved the cancer care or the pediatric part of it. So I made sure to have both experiences in the first half of my PGY1 so that I could figure out if I wanted to do a PGY2, and if so, in what specialty.

As my first elective opportunity, I scheduled one of Northwestern's multiple opportunities in cancer care. However, at the time we did not have a pediatric experience. There was a rotation available in the neonatal intensive care unit (ICU), but our hospital cared for newborns and adults, not children. We were attached to a children's hospital, so I worked with my residency director, Noelle Chapman, who created an opportunity in a pediatric ICU at the children's hospital and in the neonatal ICU at Northwestern. My experiences as a PGY1 made it evident that my passion was in hematology/oncology, not pediatrics.

In my PGY1, one of the most important things I did was find mentors and sponsors. I worked with a lot of great pharmacists and learned something from each of them, but by no means did I want to be exactly like any of them. I took parts of what each of them did and incorporated them into who I was becoming as a pharmacist. No matter how well or poorly I got along with or understood a preceptor, I still made sure to learn from what he or she did well. I took all of this plus what I learned from pharmacy speakers and my mentors and sponsors, and I shaped who I was as my patients' pharmacist.

Residency is about a lot of things, but one of them is learning who you are as a pharmacist and a professional. *While you have the opportunity to be both a pharmacist and a trainee, do the things that you find most challenging as often as you possibly can. Take opportunities that you do not necessarily feel qualified for and work hard to do them well.*

For me, my biggest challenge at the start of residency was public speaking. During college, when I spoke in front of large crowds, my face would turn bright red and the expression on my face was anything but confident. I decided to take on the challenge of public speaking during my PGY1. My first rotation was in administration with our pharmacy director, Desi Kotis, who was organizing the first Women in Pharmacy Conference at Northwestern which was scheduled for two months after my rotation. I participated in meetings about what would be discussed, who would present, etc. Noelle Chapman, who at the time was about 7 months pregnant, was scheduled to give a presentation on authentic leadership. Her due date was basically the day that she was supposed to present, so I offered to present for her. When the offer came out of my mouth, I instantly felt slightly terrified. I became the backup plan that ended up being the actual plan as she delivered a few days before the presentation. I practiced relentlessly and wore a thick coat of makeup so that no one could see my face turn the color of a cherry as I presented; I felt confident as I gave the presentation. From then on, I have continued to challenge myself and give presentations on a local and national level, so that now I feel much more confident in my ability to speak in public.

After discovering my true passion in pharmacy (hematology/oncology) and forming the basics of who I was as a pharmacist, I decided to apply to seven residencies across the country instead of early commit to Northwestern. I loved Northwestern, but I felt I had to explore outside my current institution to make sure that the PGY2 in oncology at Northwestern was what best suited me. I interviewed across the country and at Northwestern and discovered some great PGY2 programs. I even took some of those aspects and incorporated them into the program I chose.

Joe and I decided to couples match for PGY2. We had interviewed all over the country and knew that we did not want to end up with one of us in Utah and the other in North Carolina (which was a very real possibility). Ranking our PGY2s was a very different discussion than it was for PGY1. It was one of our first experiences as a couple making a huge life decision as a team. Ultimately, we both matched at Northwestern (Joe in critical care and me in oncology) and became co-residents.

Lesson learned: No matter how much you think you know about someone, you always have more to learn about them. My husband and I actually worked pretty well as co-residents and got to see each other in a whole new environment. We also planned a wedding together during our PGY2, and we both survived to walk down the aisle, which I consider to be a BIG win.

During my PGY2, I realized that our program did not have any clinically-focused required rotations in outpatient practice. We also did not have any clinical pharmacists working side-by-side with the physicians providing direct patient care in the outpatient setting. I wanted to experience outpatient practice, so I took the initiative and requested to work with the physicians in some of the clinics. My experiences took off from there; I worked with physicians and for many of them, I was their first exposure to working directly with a clinical pharmacist.

After my first clinic experience, I was pretty certain that providing direct patient care in the outpatient cancer clinics was exactly what I wanted to do for my career. However, at the end of my PGY2, there was still no clinical pharmacist in a direct patient care role in oncology at Northwestern. I looked at other institutions, but when I spoke with my PGY2 director who was also the oncology pharmacy manager, Mary Golf, she said that some physicians after working with me had requested that a pharmacist join them in clinic. Even better, the department was making plans for the position, and Mary offered me a position as one of the pharmacists to start it. I was hooked. I decided to stay at Northwestern to start a completely new service line in outpatient oncology clinical pharmacy that I had laid the foundation for during my PGY2. Another pharmacist and I started that new service, working with the gastrointestinal and skin cancer teams 6 months after I completed my PGY2.

Throughout my residency experiences and now in the early parts of my career as an oncology pharmacist, the two most important things that I have learned are as follows:

1. Surround yourself in both your professional and personal life with people who challenge and support you in pursuing your passion.

2. If a position or experience does not exist in your current environment and you want to do it, insist on creating it and work relentlessly on doing so.

I hope that my story will help you find your path, and remind you that you do not have to know exactly where you are going when you start your journey, but you should try to learn as much as you can along the way.

Chelsea

Andre D. Harvin
PharmD, MS, BCPS

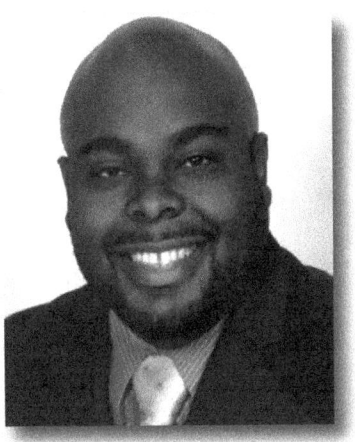

Follow Your Passions—Random Personal Encounters Provide Career Guidance

Andre reflects on a series of life-long personal encounters that have been pivotal to his professional life and his career advancement. He illustrates how various events over the years have influenced his career directions and how he still relies on such opportunities to shape his goals.

Andre is currently Pharmacy Branch Manager at OptumRx, Kernersville, North Carolina after recently serving as a Pharmacy System Manager of Inpatient Operations at Wake Forest Baptist Health in Winston Salem, North Carolina. He received a BS degree in Biochemistry from the University of Maryland, his PharmD from the University of Michigan, and completed a postgraduate year 1 (PGYI)/PGY2/MS health-system pharmacy administration residency and graduate degree program at The Ohio State University Wexner Medical Center in Columbus.

Andre's advice is: **Listen to others' advice and follow your goals with perseverance; realize opportunities are often unexpected but should always be considered; hesitancy and self-doubt are expected; and continue to reassess your own "best self."**

Dear Pharmacy Colleague,

During the first year of my first position after my residency, I was eager to impress my

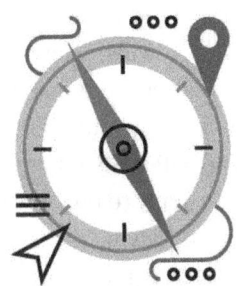

boss. I worked ridiculous hours, took on every project possible, and never took a day off. I maintained this pace for the nearly a year before a sales representative who was visiting our facility gave me some advice. He warned me about burnout and told me my current path would lead to a career-limiting decision before I knew it. I realized his advice was a wake-up call; I began to aggressively manage expectations to ensure I could deliver the quality of work I was capable of with my resources.

His advice reminds me of other career-altering encounters that have brought me to this stage of my life.

CAREER-ALTERING ENCOUNTERS

My first such encounter came along before I even knew what a pharmacist did. I was born in Baltimore, Maryland to a single-parent mother doing her best with limited resources. We didn't have much, but what we had we cherished. When I was in middle school, she read *Gifted Hands* by Ben Carson to me. The book changed my life as it was the first time a person who looked like me was notable for his intellect rather than his athletic ability or comedic timing. My admiration for Dr. Carson only grew over time as I saw a reflection of my own life in his experiences. If he could go from nearly living on the streets to being one of the greatest neurosurgeons in the world, what could I achieve with a similar mindset?

Years later, I had the opportunity to meet Dr. Carson in person. I asked him how he accomplished so much with so many barriers in his life. His response was to highlight a quote in his book:

> "Success is determined not by whether or not you face obstacles, but by your reaction to them. And if you look at these obstacles as a containing fence, they become your excuse for failure. If you look at them as a hurdle, each one strengthens you for the next."

It was a simple response, but it meant so much to me to have that interaction. What I learned from Dr. Carson is how to define one of the most important traits of a leader: **perseverance**. Anyone who has ever spent time with me and asked me about my leadership philosophy would admit that perseverance comes up multiple times. As a leader, obstacles are a guarantee; the best leaders I know face each obstacle directly and, whether they succeed or fail, they always learn from it. Having been a pharmacist for only four years at the writing of this letter, I have lost count of the number of obstacles that I have faced both personally and professionally. I would love to say that I handled each with poise but that would be a falsehood. I have tripped, stumbled, and fallen more times than I can count; after each obstacle, I collect myself, reflect, and prepare for the next one.

My next encounter came during a pivotal time in my life and lasted only a few minutes. I was approaching my senior year in undergraduate school when I desperately wondered where I was going in life. My first two years in college were marred with underachievement and frustration. Despite my rededication to my studies and improved academic performance over the following two years, my GPA was far from competitive. At the moment when I was deciding whether or not to apply to pharmacy school, fate would intervene with a chance encounter. It was Thanksgiving evening. Instead of resting on the couch with family, I was in line at the mall hoping to be one of the first patrons into an electronics store to get the Black Friday deals. While standing outside attempting to stay warm, I struck up a conversation with a gentleman that would change the course of my professional career.

After first discussing the ridiculousness of standing outside in near freezing weather for discounts on items we certainly didn't need, he began asking me questions to pass the time. I told him that I was finishing my bachelor's degree but didn't know what I wanted to do next. I admitted that my academic career hadn't panned out the way I had anticipated due to my loss of focus. As our conversation continued, he taught me another lesson that I carry with me to this day: *hesitancy and self-doubt are a part of each success story*. His advice was to embrace my failures rather than hide them. At the time the advice seemed naïve; why highlight a failure when I can enhance my strengths? I walked away from the conversation appreciative of his time, but wary of the advice.

It was almost a year later when I mustered the courage to apply to pharmacy schools. I initially decided that I would only apply to one or two programs because applications were expensive, and I could not afford to waste my funds on an opportunity that might not pan out. I narrowed my choices to local-area schools and sent in my applications early. By chance, the following week I crossed paths with the gentleman from Black Friday again. We instantly recognized each other and struck up another conversation. I told him that he should be proud because I had taken his advice and decided to apply to pharmacy school, but that I was applying only to two programs due to the cost. He implored me to invest in my own success and told me that I would never regret spending the money to further my education. He suggested that if I applied to only one additional program, I should make it count and shoot for the stars. That week I sat down and wrote my application essay to the University of Michigan College of Pharmacy; four years later I walked across the Michigan stage at The Big House with my PharmD in hand. To this day, I credit two random conversations and the kindness of a stranger with one of the greatest accomplishments of my life. Although he may never know the role he played in my life, I remember those conversations and his career advice.

My most recent encounter and final story happened very recently in my career. It challenged me to evaluate what I value in my career and question if my current path is the right one. It occurred during the hiring process for a new per diem pharmacist on my staff. There were numerous applicants, but interactions with a particular applicant resulted in playing a pivotal role in my career. At that time, I was firmly entrenched in my position, involved in numerous projects, had visibility and recognition across the organization, and was on a team I enjoyed representing on a daily basis. When I began looking through the applications, one candidate stood out. He seemed to have had experience in nearly every aspect of our profession: retail, hospital, long-term care, industry, etc. I arranged for the interview to see if he was really serious about being a per diem pharmacist when his resume suggested he had little interest in maintaining any singular role. During the interview, I expressed my concerns with his job history pattern and inquired about why he chose to move so often. His answer was that he was searching for his **best self**. After over a decade of being a pharmacist, he was still searching for the same passion that brought him to the profession for a satisfying role in patient care.

Enamored by his story, I realized it took great courage to make such drastic changes in employment, especially in a profession that prizes stability. It was after this interview that I first gave serious consideration to changing my own career path. I considered not just a new position or promotion, but how I could uniquely contribute to the delivery of care as a pharmacist. The interaction led me to consider careers outside of traditional health-system pharmacy roles. I eventually decided to make the move to pharmacy managed care practice, a completely different pharmacy practice environment. The realization that I wanted to change my practice environment has truly been enlightening. It was one of the most difficult choices I have had to make. I made the choice after finally realizing that I, too, was not living up to my **best self**. However, I am pleased that I made my decision to follow my passion. Who knows what the future will hold, but I know that if I continue to work to find my best self, I will be fulfilled in the end.

When I joined our profession, it was to be part of the most accessible and trusted health professionals in the country. Each day our individual actions impact countless patients, family members, and other medical professionals. There has never been a more challenging and yet rewarding time to be a pharmacist. A little over a decade ago, when I first decided that I wanted to pursue a career in pharmacy, the landscape was completely different and would be unrecognizable to today's new graduates.

I hope this letter not only highlights how my unexpected encounters impacted my own life but emphasizes how important it is to make every encounter or opportunity worthwhile in your career. Try ensuring that at least one person you interact with today is better because of your kind gesture, words, or actions toward them. Your impact on that person's life could be immeasurable, and you may just inspire another person to follow their passion.

Regards,

Andre

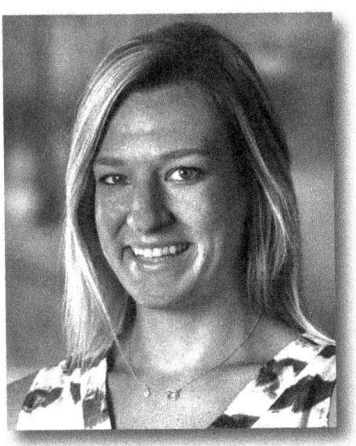

Molly Henry
PharmD

Live Life on Purpose

Molly is an uplifting, engaging, and dynamic person, pharmacist, and resident. Everyone who interacts with Molly feels the positivity radiating from her heart. She is thoughtful and caring; she lifts up others around her. Molly has quickly become the pharmacist who patients request by name and remember because of the tender care that she gives. Her personality will continue to give hope to countless others!

Molly is currently a postgraduate year 2 (PGY2) solid organ transplant pharmacy resident at Nebraska Medicine, Omaha, and completed her ASHP accredited PGY1 pharmacy residency at Nebraska Medicine. She earned her PharmD degree with distinction at University of Iowa, College of Pharmacy, Iowa City.

Molly's advice is: *Build strong relationships; know, develop, and utilize your strengths; live life on purpose; and remember attitude is key!*

Dear Pharmacy Colleague,

Like many students, I had a lot of unknowns as an 18-year-old starting my freshman year at a large university and about to embark on the next phase of my life. One thing I knew for sure was that I had a strong desire to work in healthcare. I spent the first couple years

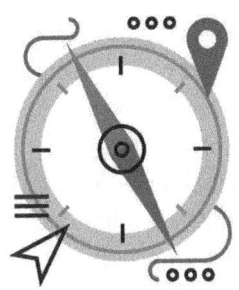

of my college career exploring a number of different careers. Just after my sophomore year, I took a leap of faith and went on a medical mission trip to Peru. I had one of those chance encounters that shaped my life forever. I spent two weeks working with a number of different healthcare providers in a unique environment. The team included physicians, surgeons, nurses, and pharmacists. For the first time, I had exposure to what an interdisciplinary team looked like and I realized that there are many ways pharmacists can impact patient care which further strengthened my interest in becoming one.

One year later I began my pharmacy school journey. I was exposed to the unique roles pharmacists have within the healthcare team and with patients. Throughout pharmacy school I remember yearning for a position where I could work alongside a team and be an advocate for my patients. Visualizing the future impact I could have on my patients inspired me to apply and complete a PGY1 residency. Throughout my PGY1 residency, I began to develop a strong interest in the solid organ transplant population. My passion for caring for these types of patients further confirmed my desire to complete a PGY2 residency in solid organ transplantation. The memories made, lessons learned, relationships formed, and the person and pharmacist I have become are all testaments to why residency has been and continues to be worth every hard-working second. I want to share a few lessons that I have learned throughout residency training and describe the impact they have had on me personally and professionally.

LESSON #1. BUILD STRONG RELATIONSHIPS

This is the most important lesson I learned. Much of the tidbits of wisdom I gained were often a result of my interactions and relationships I developed with many wonderful practitioners. As I began my PGY1 year, I anticipated that there would be many exciting unknowns. The first pleasant surprise was meeting my co-residents who would become like family to me. I remember the first day of residency orientation when I sat wide-eyed and excited as I looked around the room, and I could feel a similar sense of camaraderie among all of my co-residents. We all had our unique stories and reasons why we decided to pursue a residency. What struck me was how passionate we all were to learn and develop ourselves as pharmacists so that we could have a positive impact on patient care. The best part about the year was that many friendships developed, first as co-residents and then by the end of the year as brothers and sisters—a residency family. Each of my co-residents impacted me in a different and powerful way. There were those who impacted me throughout the daily business of residency life, and those who impacted me in the silence of my heart. What made this special was that even though we had our individual dreams and aspirations, we were all going through the ups and downs of residency training and were there for each other.

Residency also provided me with countless opportunities to strengthen relationships with my preceptors who quickly became my role models and trusted mentors. The definition of a *mentor* is an experienced and trusted advisor. Mentors will give you advice as a young practitioner, advocate as you embark on your pharmacy career, and willingly offer their time, talents, and advice to ensure your success. A mentor may be someone you reach out to *intentionally* or you develop a relationship with *naturally*. In my experience, from those naturally developed relationships were my best mentors because they had a vested interest in helping me succeed. My mentors all had one thing in common—they identified my strengths and helped me to improve upon them. The other similarity is that all of my mentors are strong advocates for me as a pharmacist and are constantly seeking out opportunities for me as a young professional. My preceptors and mentors continue to inspire me to do my best so that I will be able to impact future students and residents in the same way they have done for me. All of these relationships have had a significant effect on my life, and I will forever be grateful for the experiences I have had with each of them.

LESSON #2. KNOW, DEVELOP, AND UTILIZE YOUR STRENGTHS

During orientation, our director of pharmacy asked our residency class what strengths we each possessed. He encouraged us to know our strengths and to actively utilize them. I now realize that throughout my PGY1 year, knowing and utilizing my strengths were a large part of my success. We often think only about our weaknesses and focus on how to improve. While it is important to know your weaknesses, it is more important to know, develop, and utilize your strengths. For example, I learned early on that a strength or asset of mine is adaptability. I was encouraged to use it to enhance my relationships with patients and providers as I rotated through various experiences as a PGY1. Knowing this strength early on helped me to have a more successful residency year. By identifying my own strengths, I have been able to utilize them to contribute to the healthcare team and to become a better pharmacist for my patients.

LESSON #3. LIVE LIFE ON PURPOSE

During the first quarter of my PGY2 year, I had the opportunity to attend a residency class leadership retreat. We discussed our aspirations, communication styles, and ways to improve our leadership abilities. One presenter impressed me with his advice to "live life on purpose." He encouraged us to really know ourselves, to think of how we wanted to be remembered, and to define our own "personal brand." Not only is this an important life message, it is also important in pursuing a career. I want patients and co-workers to remember me as the pharmacist who made them feel better when they were going through a hard time, the pharmacist who went above and beyond to make their experience just a little bit better. I would encourage you to reflect on what "living life on purpose" means to you and identify what your "brand" is as you shape your career and your future.

LESSON #4. ATTITUDE IS KEY

This is an important message that I learned very quickly. Early in the morning, as I sat in my residency office with eight other residents, there was always a whirlwind of emotions floating around. All it would take was one negative interaction to affect (or infect) everyone. We all face challenges. If I had let those challenges break me down and affect my attitude, I may never have had such a fulfilling residency experience.

The truth is that residency has been one of the most challenging yet rewarding experiences of my life. There have been weeks when my lack of sleep negatively affected my attitude, and I easily could have been that negative voice in the room. However, by keeping my spirits high and remaining positive, I had a better work environment and an overall better day. For example, I remember walking into a patient's room to provide discharge education to a newly transplanted patient. I could tell that he was exhausted and worn down from the toll of the difficult journey over the past few days. I knew I would spend at least an hour with this patient, and I was determined to maintain a positive and uplifting attitude. As I continued my instruction on medication education and got to know the patient, I started to see something change in his eyes. He started asking questions and became engaged in conversation, and I could hear hope in his voice. When I completed my educational discussion, the patient feverishly thanked me for spending my afternoon with him. In that moment, I realized that my attitude may have made this patient feel better and given him hope during a difficult time. It is experiences like these that remind me why I do what I do and why ATTITUDE is so important.

These experiences are just the beginning of (what I hope to be) a very long and fulfilling pharmacy career. My residency experience has taught me how to be a better pharmacist, introduced me to some of the most influential people of my career, and propelled me into a fast-paced and ever changing profession. I will always be evolving the way I think, the way I work with my team, and the way I care for my patients. Residency has been the trampoline that I have utilized to jump high into my professional career. My residency experiences have given me the background knowledge, confidence, and desire for life-long learning.

As you consider your own residency journey, my hope is that you take advantage of as many wonderful opportunities as you are able and use them as stepping stones to help you achieve your goals, dreams, and aspirations. *Now go out and "live your life with a purpose!"*

Best wishes,

Molly

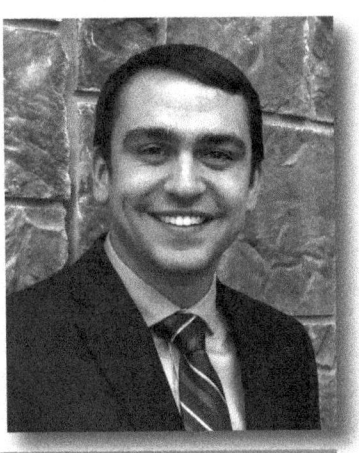

Brian Kempin
PharmD, MS

Mentors Are the Key to Success—Residency in the Rearview Mirror

Brian credits his successful residency selection, training, and now his career beginnings to several influential mentors. He sought out a variety of mentors starting in his first year of pharmacy school to help direct his career path.

Brian is currently Manager, Clinical Operations, at the University of Virginia Health System, in Charlottesville. He received his PharmD at the University of Kansas and his postgraduate year 1 (PGY1)/PGY2 MS health-system pharmacy administration (HSPA) residency from the University of Virginia Health System in Charlottesville.

Brian's advice is: *Be present. Before you leave work each day, walk through the offices and see what people are working on and ask questions. Get involved in their projects; this will help build your experiences and decision making skills.*

Dear Pharmacy Colleague,

I can now say, without hesitation, that I am confidently pursuing the most fitting pharmacy career path for my talents and interests. However, I wasn't always certain what career path I wanted to pursue within the pharmacy profession. When I look in

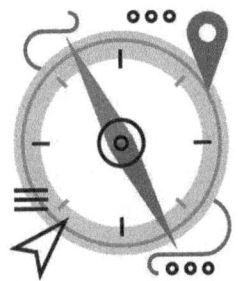

my rearview mirror, I am convinced that without the presence of influential mentors my pharmacy career would look much different. When the time comes to start evaluating your career options as a pharmacist, look no further than one who has gone down the same path before you. I can say with assurance that mentorship has been the key to my success in determining the direction I wanted to pursue in the pharmacy world.

During my first year as a pharmacy student, I obtained an internship at a hospital and was privileged to work with leaders in the field who saw potential in me and wanted to maximize my impact within the profession. Their willingness to teach and inspire the next generation, while taking time out of their schedules, was influential in my future career decisions. I was able to have discussions about pharmacy career pathways for both clinical and administrative residencies. It was over breaks in my internship that my mentor inspired me to create short- and long-term goals for my professional career.

At this time, I also acquired an immense amount of information on pros and cons for each residency type through my mentor sharing his past experience. During the three-year-long internship and relationship with my mentors, it became evident to me that I wanted to pursue a health-system pharmacy administration residency that would also provide advanced clinical training and learning opportunities. I then looked at specific residency programs that would help me achieve my goals of having a global impact on patients and advancing the practice of pharmacy.

MAKING SHORT- AND LONG-TERM GOALS TO GUIDE YOUR WAY

Analyzing the many outstanding organizations that offered a health-system pharmacy administration residency was my next challenge. In examining the residency programs, I was struggling to decide which program was best for me. Fortunately my mentor encouraged me to revert back to the short- and long-term goals that I had created and to use them as a lens to look through when reviewing the programs. Using those goals as a guideline, I was able to see what residency programs aligned best with my determined purpose and career path. The programs offered at the ASHP Midyear Clinical Meeting made me realize *many* programs had excellent learning opportunities to help me achieve my short- and long-term goals. In addition to the experiences I would receive at the residency site, my mentor recommended that I also evaluate the programs based on the learning environment and the personal fit within the program. I remember my mentor saying, "*You don't want to go to a residency site where you can't be yourself for two years.*" Alignment of goals and personal fit were the driving factors that helped me in assessing which programs to apply to for an onsite interview.

When it came time to rank the residency programs, I wanted a program that would push me out of my comfort zone, expand my clinical skills, and advance my administrative knowledge and decision-making. I wanted a program where I could see the potential to advance from a learner to a leader in the department. It wasn't until onsite interviews that I was able to see the passion of the program from discussions with the directors. One of the program directors really inspired me to pursue my career at that organization when he said, "*In this residency we will push you to occasionally fail, but you will fail in a safe environment that will teach you to learn from your mistakes and ensure that the next time you will have the experience to make a more appropriate decision.*" I was strongly encouraged and impressed that the program would instill enough trust in me to stand behind my decisions, right or wrong, and wanted to help me advance. Undoubtedly, I knew the program would invest in me and provide the hands-on experience I would need to help me be successful post-residency. This experience, together with the advice from my mentor, enabled me to envision my short- and long-term goals coming to fruition at that program—it was a place where I could be myself and grow.

After Match Day comes and goes, you would think the rest of the road would be a straight shot to where I am today. But there are many paths and possibilities that require experience to navigate. However, certain approaches can help you make the most of your years in residency and gain that experience. One approach was passed on to me before I left to travel halfway across the country to begin my first year of residency. My mentor told me, "*Be present. Before you leave each day, walk through the offices and see what people are working on and ask questions. Get involved in their projects; this will help build your experiences and your decision making skills.*" If you just put your head down and don't look around to take in all of the learning opportunities, you will undoubtedly miss out on valuable experiences that help you get the most out of your residency. The learning opportunities that come from unplanned and spontaneous experiences can far exceed your list of residency requirements. Since completing my residency I can say that being present in the moment played an important role in my learning experience, and this advice allowed me to get the most out of my residency.

REMEMBER TO BALANCE YOUR LIFE

During residency you will surely face challenges and uphill battles that could cause you to burn out and lose sight of your short- and long-term goals. I found it critical to refocus on my goals to reignite my motivation and obtain a "second wind" to complete the task in front of me. However, for lasting success, it was equally important to learn how to leave work *at* work. Understanding that deadlines are important and managing your time is a key to success; however, if you continue to view emails, work on projects, or can't put a continuing education book down after your day ends, you will miss life moments you will never be able to get back. This will result in a hindrance of your success and the possibility of permanently losing sight of your goals.

My perspective on work–life integration changed in January of my PGY2 year when my wife and I were blessed with the birth of our daughter. I quickly realized that there are greater moments than pharmacy accomplishments or minor issues that can be resolved the next day. If all you are doing and thinking about is pharmacy, you should do a self-check of your personal goals to make sure you do not expend all your energy at work and then don't make time for yourself and those around you.

It was easy for me to be in the moment and forget to lift my head up for a breath outside of pharmacy. However, I am fortunate to have a loving and supportive wife who reminded me to take breaks and enjoy opportunities outside pharmacy. These moments actually rejuvenated my energy, and I was able to pick back up where I had left off with my pharmacy tasks. Ensuring that your personal and professional goals are compatible and can both be achieved is crucial in preventing burnout during residency and beyond.

Selecting the right path that maximizes your talents within the profession of pharmacy is not an easy task. I strongly encourage building a relationship with a mentor who has been in the profession for several years and informed about multiple pharmacy career pathways. Be vigilant from the beginning with your short- and long term goals and always revert back to your road map of those goals when making life decisions within the profession. When the time arises that you may need to revise your road map, it is fine to seek out mentorship in blazing a new trail. Remember, comfort may not always be the best option when it comes to what is best for your professional career, and the balance between professional and personal life is key to your overall success.

Make each decision with bold intentions and self-confidence, knowing that each accomplishment brings you closer to achieving your goals.

Brian

Patryk Kornecki
PharmD

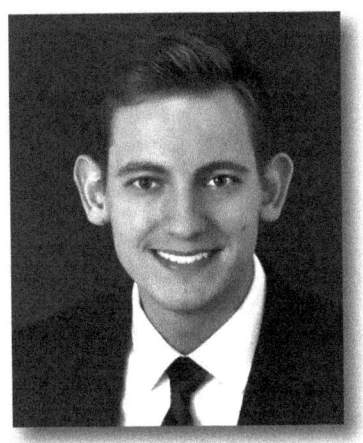

Reasons to Do a Residency, How to Select the Right One, and How to Maximize Its Value

Patryk is a motivated, passionate, and versatile pharmacist who embraces his experiences with Walgreens community and local specialty/health-system pharmacies to lead, enhance, and redefine the practice of pharmacy for his team and patients. He is known for providing excellent patient care and communications as well as teaching in a variety of healthcare and academic settings.

Patryk is currently a Walgreens Local Specialty Pharmacist in Boston, Massachusetts. He completed an accredited community pharmacy residency at Walgreens Specialty and Northeastern University in Boston, having received his PharmD from the Massachusetts College of Pharmacy and Health Sciences in Boston.

Patryk's advice is: *Take chances on new experiences because it will give you confidence to make important decisions later on. It was because of the chances and challenges I took early that I could cross paths with fantastic mentors, difficult patients, and new environments.*

Dear Pharmacy Colleague,

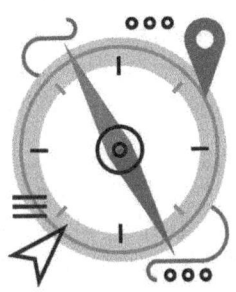

It was a cold autumn night when my pharmacist drove me home after a successful closing shift. We both reflected on our day and set the bar higher for the next. After exchanging thoughts and excitement about the good work our team does, he asked me, "Patryk ... have you thought of doing a residency program with Walgreens?" And so the seed was planted.

As a senior in high school and student in college, I was always passionate about community pharmacy and the ability to change people's lives. I started my relationship with Walgreens as a volunteer intern through high school in Clifton, New Jersey. Immediately, I became inspired by the work we did and the role we played in our community.

I set my first goal: To become an intern for Walgreens. The following year, however, our company faced a hiring freeze. Keeping the dream alive, I began a series of many email exchanges with my pharmacy supervisor that ultimately resulted in a stronger relationship. In the years that followed, I worked at many different Walgreen pharmacies in the New Jersey and Boston regional areas, gaining experience and meeting fantastic people along the way.

The following are a few important traits that I think are important.

BE PERSISTENT

I visualize persistence as knocking on the doors of opportunity. As a young professional student, it's difficult to develop a sense of confidence early on, but persistence in your goals and dreams will certainly get you there. It is also reassuring to know that a lack of persistence was not the cause of your failures. Reflecting back on my journey, persistence served as the foundation for developing greater confidence and the ability to overcome adversity during difficult times. This very same characteristic helped me gain my first shift at a specialty pharmacy. I was tenacious and kept asking for new experiences and opportunities. That pharmacy later became the site of my residency program. People around you will notice your persistence as it shows you have ambition; when demonstrated professionally and diplomatically, it also shows initiative.

BE OPEN

The ability to take chances on new experiences gave me confidence to make important decisions. The chances and challenges I took early in my career enabled me to cross paths with fantastic mentors, difficult patients, and new environments. It is important to begin a journey of self-reflection and analyze your own strengths, weaknesses, likes, and dislikes. Each experience and encounter had an impact on my personal and professional growth, painting a clearer picture of who I wanted to become and where I wanted to be. You, too, can be an artist, but it has to start with being open and then reflecting on those new experiences. Steve Jobs remarked that, "You can't connect the dots looking forward; you can only connect them looking backwards. So you have to trust that the dots will somehow connect in your future."

I committed to pursuing a residency program because I wanted to be a part of momentous change, be on the cusp of innovation, and help push the boundaries of community pharmacy. Most importantly, I wanted to take my experiences with patient care a level deeper. The benefits of completing a residency program that I hadn't recognized until its culmination were exponential growths in leadership, preceptorship, and craftsmanship. Especially valuable was the time spent under the guidance of preceptors, the daily feedback, and dynamic change from day to day and month to month.

My original thought of pursuing a community residency program came with some hesitation as these are still relatively new areas of growth. What I failed to realize was the high level of expertise needed in the niche of specialty pharmacy. As a resident, I worked at the bedside with patients undergoing solid organ and bone marrow transplants and assisted with the clinical care for patients receiving oral chemotherapy, infectious disease, and autoimmune treatments. The ability to assist and advocate for patients in gaining access to medication at what may be the most fragile point of their lives is privileging, yet humbling at the same time. I relay these experiences because of the effect and importance of placing oneself in unfamiliar situations. It allows you to discover new opportunities and interests. Throughout the course of my program, I've witnessed transformation and growth, slowly being pushed outside the bird's nest and able to fly. The characteristics of persistence and openness have proven essential to my journey.

Many residency programs have an academic component associated with them. As somebody who is passionate about teaching students, I had the opportunity to facilitate weekly seminar sessions, participate in pharmacy laboratories, and serve as a role model and resource. Close collaboration with my academic preceptor has given me the skills to become a better mentor for students and a better presenter at national conferences. I value the time my mentors dedicated to me during my journey early on, and believe it is intrinsic to return the gift.

Two traits—personal values, really—I found most impactful throughout my invested year in residency training are the abilities to be humble and to value humanity.

BE HUMBLE

A cornerstone to success and a willingness to learn come with being humble. As students, we have a constant drive for success, which the competitive nature of school breeds in us. However, it's important to stay grounded and turn those emotions into productive actions, or else the mind becomes inhibited to new thoughts and turns stagnant. Staying humble extends beyond our immediate pharmacy team and applies to everybody around us: patients, classmates, friends, and family. *I've discovered that each person I have come across in life serves a valuable purpose and lesson*, and it's important to keep that thought at the heart of our work and actions, every day.

BE HUMAN

It was Rebecca Shanahan, President of the National Association of Specialty Pharmacy, who reinforced (at the conference in Washington, DC in 2017) that despite all of the great advancements and growth in specialty pharmacy, we must always value humanity and keep it at the core of our work, every day. This serves as a reminder that despite dynamic change and progression, the core of everyday work must revolve around the greater good for the patient. If you practice this daily, then you provide value to your work and build trusting relationships with patients and those around you.

Reflecting back, I'm able to connect the dots in my life to move forward. The foundational characteristics of persistence and openness have intertwined with humbleness and humanity, each stepping stone building genuine character.

Moving forward, how do you choose a residency program and what are the next steps?

Research is critical to making the right decision; being open and taking a chance then follows that important moment. The residency coordinator for all Walgreens programs, Judy Sommers-Hanson, always said that if you've seen one specialty pharmacy, then you've seen only one specialty pharmacy. Each program you come across during your research is unique, situated in a different area, and influenced by specific cultures. Understanding the offerings of each program is the beginning of your work— then, differentiate unique experiences (health-system versus community, academic focus versus clinical, urban versus suburban location). Lastly, be open and knock on some doors; contacting or meeting residency program directors and current residents will bring greater perspective to your decision-making process and show interest. Not everything can be answered through a brochure or web site description. Getting to the source of knowledge will be valuable and offer greater insight.

Once your research phase is completed, meeting directors and residents at the ASHP Midyear Clinical Meeting will allow them to connect emotion between your curriculum vitae and application. Perhaps fate will have it that you discover other programs and people of interest while networking. I find conferences to be one of the most dynamic ways of sharing knowledge, meeting interesting leaders, and re-inspiring the pharmacy community of our unified progression. As your application files close and interview invitations begin, preparation will be the key to success. Each site will have its unique interview process; preparing for each using your initial and continued research allows for a level of personalization and understanding. It's important to use specific examples and reference some of the best experiences of your journey up until this point. Then, future resident, you can celebrate your success come Match Day and know that fate has chosen the right program for you!

I am confident that I would not have had the opportunities this early in my career if it was not for my preceptors' invested time with me during residency training. It's true that one year of residency is equivalent to a few years of practice as the level of integration is deep and structured. Most importantly, starting your career on the right path under supportive leadership and preceptorship only multiplies your growth and future success. For me, it was Roy Youn—the pharmacist, mentor, and friend—who changed the direction of my post-graduate career and opened the door to new possibilities. I owe a great deal in return to all of the mentors who have chiseled my thoughts and experiences to what they are today.

Good luck, future resident, on your journey to discovery, learning, and growth to make a difference in your community and the lives around you.

Patryk

Noelle Lee
PharmD

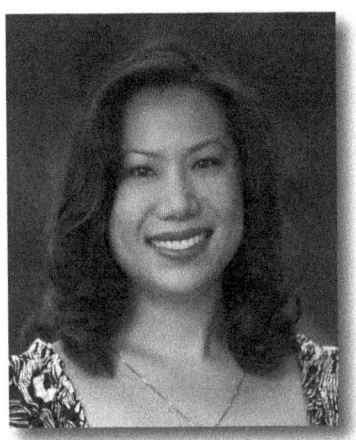

Find Joy in What You Do, Identify Personal Expectations, and Continue Learning

Noelle relates to people and senior leaders at every level of her organization. Last year Noelle's chief executive officer (CEO) chose her as one of three front-line staff to be interviewed in front of 2,000 managers, directors, and vice-presidents about her experiences as a new employee. The most important qualities that everyone searches for in their staff—character, integrity, and optimism—describe Noelle as a person, resident, and now as a pharmacist.

Noelle is currently Pharmacy Benefit Coordinator, Sutter Health System Office, Sacramento, California. She completed her postgraduate year 1 (PGY1) accredited pharmacy residency at the Sutter Health System Office, Sacramento, California. Noelle received her PharmD degree at the University of California San Francisco and her BS degree at the University of California San Diego.

Noelle's advice is: *Remember to give back. Participate in professional pharmacy associations, serve as a preceptor, or volunteer as a mentor. I guarantee you will be rewarded ten-fold, knowing that you have not only contributed to the field of pharmacy, but you have also sustained the legacy of our profession.*

Dear Pharmacy Colleague,

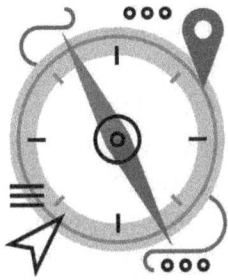

I pursued an ASHP PGY1 pharmacy practice residency because I viewed it as a necessity for my professional development as a pharmacist—a perspective that is specific to my story. As a pharmacy student, I focused mainly on research, which limited my pharmacy practice rotations. My hope was that from a PGY1 program, I would gain invaluable experience working in a variety of pharmacy settings, one of which would be the launch point of my career. My concern was that if I entered the workforce directly after pharmacy school, the opportunity to pursue a residency mid-career would not be possible. I learned later that this was an unfounded fear. It is never too late to pursue a postgraduate program. We need to remind ourselves that continued learning is essential in any profession. This is especially true for pharmacy, as evidenced by the pharmacist's ever-changing and expanding role in healthcare. Your continued education may take you beyond the clinical scope of pharmacy. After residency, I completed additional graduate coursework in healthcare analytics. By gaining knowledge in this area, I am able to interpret data both as a clinician and an analyst to identify measurable outcomes and drive efficiencies in the managed care setting.

PHARMACY SCHOOL AND DISCOVERING THE PATH FORWARD

Throughout my time at University of California San Francisco (UCSF) School of Pharmacy, I participated in student leadership, community outreach, and clinical research. However, after four years of pharmacy school, I still felt that there was much to learn and experience. I strongly believed that a postgraduate program offered me the chance to explore facets of pharmacy beyond what I had learned.

Self-reflection was critical in my decision to apply for residency and my program selection. I identified my expectations for what I wanted to get out of a residency, and weighed my preferences for each program.

Before pharmacy school, I worked as an analytical chemist in small-molecule pharmacokinetic research. Additionally, as part of my UCSF program, I was able to conduct Parkinson's disease research in zebrafish models. I wanted to build on my solid background in research. All ASHP-accredited residency programs have a longitudinal research component, so I felt drawn to this aspect of residency.

My favorite student rotation was pain management at UCSF Medical Center, where I worked mainly on arthroplasty cases. At the start of the rotation, I rarely spoke up on morning rounds with the orthopedic attendings and interns, but as the weeks went by, I found my stride. As a pharmacist in training, my role was to act as an intermediary between the patient and the physicians. I developed a much closer relationship with the patients. I spoke with patients often throughout the day, conducting pain assessments, providing medication consultations, and educating patients about anticoagulation treatment upon discharge. I enjoyed working as an active member of collaborative, interprofessional teams. By the end of the rotation, I was making recommendations to pain management and orthopedic specialists, and they respectfully heeded my advice. This was a turning point for me as a student pharmacist. I witnessed how we can break down traditional silos in healthcare. Nurses, pharmacists, physicians, case managers, and physical therapists were all working together toward the same goal of providing excellent patient care. I thrived in this environment, so I sought out a residency program that offered additional acute care experience.

Another area that I wanted to explore further was ambulatory care, as I only had one student rotation in that setting. It was important that I join a program with a residency director and preceptors who could provide support, but were also willing to promote autonomy and critical-thinking. The more I reflected and learned about myself and the variety of programs available, the more I reaffirmed my commitment to pursuing a residency program. I eventually concluded that I was looking for a balanced residency that offered a mix of research and both acute and ambulatory care rotations.

If you choose to commit yourself to a residency, identify your personal expectations. Find programs that meet your expectations, so that when you enter into a residency you are motivated to invest your time and best efforts. When you walk away from that residency, you will be proud and surprised at having accomplished so much.

I was fortunate to match with a program that far exceeded my expectations. I attribute my successful residency match to the UCSF faculty and fellow classmates, who recommended me to the program. They recognized that the Sutter Health System Office PGY1 pharmacy practice residency would provide the exact environment I sought. The program not only offered rotations in acute and ambulatory care, but also offered unique rotations in pharmacy administration and managed care. I believe my program is a rarity because not all PGY1 residencies incorporate such diverse rotations. During residency, I worked on projects such as developing pharmacist-driven protocols, performing drug use evaluations, and presenting formulary management initiatives. I valued the opportunity to implement these deliverables system-wide. I encourage you to seek out projects that allow you to work at the health-system level, rather than at a single hospital or pharmacy. This was a dynamic element of my residency that required me to communicate with clinical and administrative leadership, building my confidence and empowering me as a young pharmacist.

As I progressed through residency, I did not anticipate that my initial hope of finding the launch point of my career would stem from a four-week managed care elective. During this rotation, I worked at the Sutter Health commercial health plan, Sutter Health Plus (SHP). In my four years of pharmacy school, I had no previous exposure to managed care, and I had not participated in activities hosted by the Academy of Managed Care Pharmacy. However, in this brief, four-week rotation, I developed a strong interest and understanding of managed care concepts. I learned about pharmacy benefit manager oversight, budget impact modeling, and the impact of the Affordable Care Act. I discovered that I was able to apply various strengths and skill sets gained in other settings. For example, I utilized my analytical research skills to assess population health. I found myself working on interprofessional teams, through case management and disease management work, not unlike my acute care rotations. I was so drawn to learning more about managed care that I selected a managed care longitudinal research project, which I later presented at the Western States Conference. Again, I must attribute the next steps in my pharmacy career to sound guidance from my preceptors. They propelled me forward with their selfless support and positive reinforcement. I was fortunate to have a managed care preceptor who fostered and recognized my ability to excel in this seemingly nontraditional field of pharmacy. His optimistic energy and passion for serving as a patient advocate through clinical, managed care pharmacy is awe-inspiring. I am glad to say that this preceptor remains a trusted mentor and colleague. As my residency drew to a close, opportunity beckoned in the form of a Pharmacy Benefit Coordinator position at SHP.

I encourage you to find joy in whatever you decide to do. I look forward to coming into work every day, knowing that I am focused on providing high-quality, affordable healthcare coverage. I take great pride in the work that I do. Although I may not have a patient-facing role, I have an equally significant impact on the patient experience. The main source of my happiness is the team I work with. They are reliable friends and motivational teammates. It is important to surround yourself with people who will push you to be better and build you up. Behind every job or leadership position I have held, a mentor or peer has supported me in pursuing it. Negative relationships are toxic. I have always been a proponent of taking the good and leaving the bad, and I apply this philosophy to relationships as well.

I am humbly confident that what has brought me to this point in my career was part luck and part perseverance. It seems cliché, but it holds true for me. I am deeply grateful for the good fortune I have had. It is easy for opportunities to go unrecognized at the time they present themselves. Opportunity often wears a guise—of something fun and interesting, or sometimes of something more akin to hard work. When I started as student leader, I would not have predicted being active in professional associations beyond school. Yet, I thankfully serve on various committees within the California Pharmacists Association and as a delegate for the American Pharmacists Association. When I started my residency, I would not have predicted becoming a managed care pharmacist. Yet, I am proudly coordinating the pharmacy benefit for a budding health plan that has since seen exponential membership growth and success. We cannot anticipate the next hidden opportunity. We can only continually strive to meet our full potential, and in hindsight, identify these opportunities as milestones on our path toward self-improvement.

My last bit of advice for you is to remember to give back. Participate in professional pharmacy associations, serve as a preceptor, or volunteer as a mentor. I guarantee you will be rewarded ten-fold, knowing that you have not only contributed to the field of pharmacy, but you have also sustained the legacy of our profession.

Wishing you all the best,

Noelle

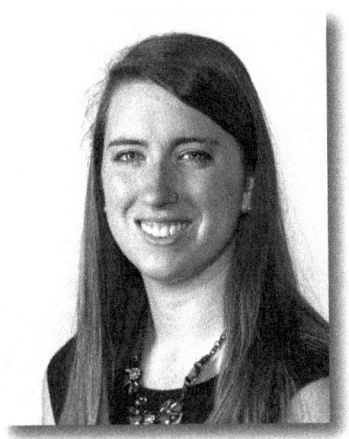

Carolyn A. Magee
PharmD

Early Planning Sets Your Career Course

Carolyn initially assumed she would be a community pharmacist. However, all that changed when she experienced a critical care advanced pharmacy practice experience (APPE) PharmD rotation. From this insightful experience, she set her career goals to pursue a postgraduate year 1 (PGY1) and PGY2 residency in this clinical direction. She then methodically planned her steps for a successful residency and career.

Carolyn is currently the Medical Surgical Intensive Care Unit (ICU) Clinical Pharmacy Specialist at the Medical University of South Carolina (MUSC). She received her Bachelor of Science in Pharmaceutical Studies from the University of Kansas and her PharmD from the University of Kansas School of Pharmacy. Carolyn completed her PGY1 pharmacy residency and PGY2 critical care pharmacy residency at University of Kentucky HealthCare, Lexington.

Carolyn's advice is: *Utilize seven tips for early career decision making: pursue your passion, make a list of non-negotiables, follow your gut, pick what is right for you, find a support system, find a mentor you trust, and get involved.*

Dear Pharmacy Colleague,

The beginning of your career is full of questions and decisions. Do you want to do a residency and, if so, where? Do you then want to follow with a PGY2 residency? Should you 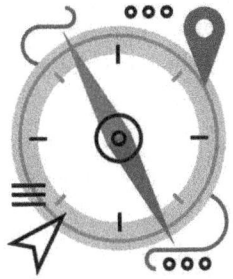 early commit to the subsequent residency? How are you going to manage the stress of residency? What kind of career do you want to pursue after residency? Where do you want to look for potential positions? What is most important to you early in your career? How are you going to set yourself on the right path? Although I cannot answer all of these questions for you, I want to share what helped me make some of these decisions.

When I started pharmacy school, I had no idea that pharmacists worked in hospitals. As an undergraduate, I took a job at a retail pharmacy and decided that was what I wanted to do with my life. However, when I completed the critical care didactic module in our last semester of pharmacy school, I found myself so engaged in the curriculum and so fascinated by the complexities involved in the care of critically ill patients that I began to see this specialty as a potential career path. My passion continued to develop on my APPE rotations. My very first rotation was in a medical intensive care unit (ICU) and I loved every second of it. Each patient was sick yet uniquely different from the patient in the next room. Although I had begun exploring the idea of residency in my last two years of pharmacy school, it was then that I ultimately decided I wanted to do a residency. This leads me to my **rule #1** for making early career decisions: **Pursue your passion**.

Finding the residency you want can be stressful. The number of options to choose from was overwhelming. I did not know how to even begin narrowing my selections. A mentor advised: **make a list of non-negotiables,** which became my **rule #2** for early career decision making. *Are you geographically limited? Are you interested in a certain specialty? Do you want a heavy emphasis in teaching? Do you want a big or small program?* For me, that meant finding programs that offered PGY2s in solid organ transplant and critical care, my two interests at the time. I pursued PGY1 residencies that had experts in these specialty areas, an affiliation with a college of pharmacy to allow for teaching opportunities, and a program that stressed learning how to be an independent clinician. My *non-negotiables* may be totally different than yours, and that is OK! This list is meant to be individualized to your specific needs. I started with a list of all of the programs that also had PGY2s in my desired specialties and weaned the number down by using my non-negotiables. The ASHP Clinical Midyear Meeting helps you further investigate the programs on your list. I prioritized speaking with the residents from those programs because they were in the shoes that I was soon to fill. I wanted to ensure they were getting the residency experience they wanted and were happy with their decision.

I remember stressing over residency applications and worrying about not getting interviews. This led me to over-applying. I ended up interviewing at 11 programs, which was entirely too many. This led to a stressful month full of interviews. I spent the entire month of February in hotel rooms and on planes and was completely exhausted. I also feel like I ended up interviewing at programs that did not fully meet my list of non-negotiables. Looking back, I wish I would have been a little more selective—it would have eliminated undue stress. Then it came time to rank programs. I separated the programs into my top picks, programs I would be happy with, and then those that I did not feel would give me the experience I wanted. I chose not to rank the programs in that last category. My top three programs were a tie in my mind; they all met my non-negotiables. I felt that each of those programs would help me develop into an independent clinician and provide the residency experience that I wanted. In the end, rather than agonizing over which to rank first, second, or third, I went with my **rule #3** of career decision making: **Go with your gut.** I chose the program that just felt the most right for me.

That ended up being one of the best decisions I had ever made. I matched for my PGY1 at the University of Kentucky (UK) HealthCare. I was nervous and yet excited to complete UK's residency program. Upon beginning my residency, the PGY1 program director corrected my thinking. He told me that *I was not there to complete the UK residency program; I was there to complete Carolyn Magee's residency program.* It was exactly this attitude that made me want to early commit for my PGY2 residency in critical care. I felt that the PGY2 program at UK was going to give me an individualized experience that pushed me in the ways I needed to be pushed. As you may have heard, there are pros and cons to early committing. One of the downsides is that I was exposed only to one healthcare system's way of doing things. But to me, the individualized experience, support from my preceptors and co-residents, and opportunities to teach and do research outweighed the potential downsides. To make this decision, I went with **rule #4** of career decision making: **Do what is right for you.** What is "right" for me may not be the same for you or any other person. If you need a change of scenery, take it. If you know a PGY2 is not right for you, seek other opportunities. Take the time to think about what is important to you and go with it.

Residency is possibly one of the most difficult things I have ever experienced. It's physically and emotionally challenging. You work long hours and have many sleepless nights. I sometimes chuckle at the concept of "work–life balance." My co-residents and I used to joke that in residency, this doesn't exist, so we coined the term *work–life integration.* Work becomes so much of your life during residency that it seems like at times they are one in the same. The only way to make it through residency is to use my **rule #5** of career decision making: **Find a support system.** I found that in my co-residents. We created this unique bond and understood each other in a way that I almost cannot explain. We supported each other through personal and professional hardships and successes. We understood what each other were going through. The root of this common bond was loving what we do—taking care of patients. Your support system does not necessarily have to be your colleagues. Others have found support from family, church communities, sports groups, and other organizations. *The most important part is having people around you who help to keep you happy and sane.*

The search for my first "real job" wasn't quite as easy as my search for a residency. I found myself feeling conflicted between faculty positions and clinical positions. On one hand, I love research and teaching; but, on the other, I learn so much from my patients and ultimately they are what drive my research curiosity and my passion for teaching. I ended up looking for both types of positions to see what was available. I found myself, like many of my peers, stressed about the entire process. It was the timing of finding a job; however, that was the most stressful. You have to start thinking about positions in November, if not earlier, even though many institutions won't know if they'll have positions open until several months later. Once you manage that hurdle, there is the timing of position offers. Do you accept the first offer or continue to pursue other positions you are interested in, but which have a delayed timeline? To help me through the stressful decision of choosing my first job I used **rule #6** for early career decision making: **Find a mentor you trust.** I was lucky to have multiple mentors that helped put things in perspective. I found it especially helpful to have a mentor in my chosen field of critical care. I used my PGY2 critical care program director, PGY1 and PGY2 advisors, who are all critical care pharmacists, as my sounding boards for choosing my first "big girl" job. They knew the job market and had an excellent understanding of the pros and cons of each position option. Although mentors in my specialty were especially helpful for me, you can find great mentors in other areas as well. Sometimes a mentor outside of pharmacy can provide more of a global "life" perspective. In the end, though, the decision is yours and yours alone.

After accepting my career position as the Medical–Surgical ICU Clinical Pharmacy Specialist at MUSC, I'm now faced with the decision of how I want to start my career. *What do I want to prioritize? What goals do I have for myself? What do I want my "mark" to be?* I'm still figuring this one out, but so far I've come up with **rule #7** for early career decision making: **Get Involved**. Really dig in to patient care. Take ownership of your role in every way that you can. Build relationships with other healthcare providers. I have decided to prioritize involvement in professional and institutional organizations because I am a firm believer in that you cannot complain about something unless you are willing to sit at the table where decisions are made. I also firmly believe that involvement at the institutional, local, and national levels is an excellent way to advance your career. I encourage each of you to really think about what is important for you and your career. *How do you want to start out? What do you want your mark to be? No matter what it is, commit to it fully.*

You have made tough decisions in the past, and you will do so in the future. I hope sharing my experiences helps you know that you are not alone when you feel stressed and overwhelmed about making decisions. Hopefully, at least one of these tips proves useful in your decision making process.

I wish you the best of luck in starting your career as a pharmacist.

Warmly,

Carolyn

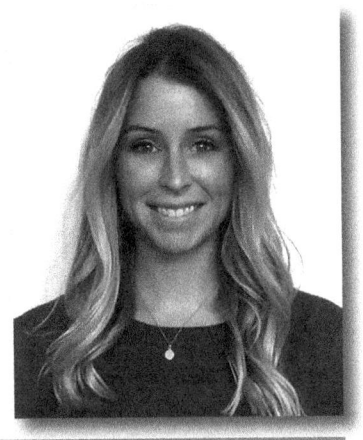

Kelley McGinnis
PharmD, MS

Analyzing Your Endless Pharmacy Career Options

Kelley started her education and training in search of her perfect career, but the options were endless—science degree, nutrition graduate degree, pharmacy degree, residencies (postgraduate year 1 [PGY1] and PGY2), or practice. She shares how she ultimately found her fulfilling career through a series of choices.

Kelley is currently an Inpatient Clinical Pharmacist in the Medical–Surgical and Emergency Department at Nebraska Medicine in Omaha. Kelley received both her BS degree in Biomedical Sciences and her MS in Nutrition at Texas A&M University at College Station. She received her PharmD at Texas Tech University Health Sciences Center School of Pharmacy in Dallas. She then completed her ASHP-accredited PGY1 residency at Nebraska Medical Center in Omaha.

Kelley's advice is: **Continue to investigate your options until your career is right for you.**

Dear Pharmacy Colleague,

As a resident, you are pulled in a thousand different directions, have more responsibilities than you know how to manage, and get far too little sleep. It's exhausting, but after you finish your residency, you'll feel like you'll have more time than you know what to do with.

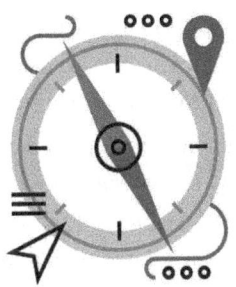

This letter will hopefully speak to those who don't have it all figured out yet. And for those who do, here's a little reminder that it's OK if things don't always go as planned, but that may be a good thing. Your interests may change significantly over the next few years. Stay open to new opportunities! As for me, there were three pivotal points in my education that ultimately landed me in my current position—a job I love where work is never "work." As a student I took a few detours on my way to pharmacy school, as a resident I struggled with the decision to early commit for a PGY2 residency, and as a professional I wanted to land the perfect first career position.

YOU DON'T KNOW WHAT YOU DON'T KNOW—CHOOSING A RESIDENCY

I was not the student that had my life goals mapped out from the beginning. I did not have the traditional childhood dream of being a veterinarian or a teacher or a doctor, but I knew I wanted to walk out of a hospital after work every day. Eventually that came to fruition, but I've lost track of the number of times I wavered on a pharmacy career. I committed to a science degree right away and put all my energy into being a successful college student with the help of bottomless coffees (Red Bulls if I am being completely honest), and spent so much time at the library I felt as though I owed them rent. Three years into my science degree, I still hadn't found my niche, but I figured pharmacy was worth consideration given my family's not-so-subtle hints about the importance of job security. I submitted pharmacy applications but almost immediately found myself second-guessing that career path. Retail pharmacy was all I knew, and I wasn't quite sure that would suit me. I applied to a master's program in nutrition instead, thinking a career as a dietitian would give me the opportunity to work closely with patients. The program was fantastic, but in the back of my mind I still wondered what kind of career I saw for my future.

Half way through graduate school, I met a mentor while on a volunteer project in a last attempt to explore pharmacy. She was a critical care pharmacist, and she asked me to take over a new research project she was working on in the intensive care unit. I realized very quickly this was a great fit and from that point on, I was completely on board with pharmacy. What other profession has opportunities ranging from retail to inpatient care to management, not to mention the dozens of other pharmacy specialties? It was another detour in my career path, but I applied and was accepted.

Fast forward to my final year (P4) in pharmacy school when residency is the topic of every conversation and deadlines are approaching fast. A large part of me wanted to start my career, make money, and avoid the looming presentations and group residency interviews. But I went in with an open mind eager to see what each program had to offer and how it would fit my interests. Several months and half a dozen flights later, I submitted my residency program rankings. I woke up early to a call from my new director on Match Day and could not have been more excited. This was the start of one of my most challenging years, but I have never once regretted that decision.

My point of this long-winded story is that your goals may evolve, and you will be given plenty of options to take a different route along the way. *Invest the time into finding what is right for you, and don't lose sight of what you want to achieve. Whether you took a victory lap in college, took time off to start a family, or started out in another field, there is no time wasted if those choices lead you to job satisfaction and success.*

PGY2 RESIDENCY OR STARTING PRACTICE—CALLING IT QUITS

As if residency wasn't hard enough, you next have to comb through potential PGY2 program descriptions, write your applications, create another presentation for interviews, and pray that when you wake up the next morning you will feel functional enough to be productive. Pivotal point number two might come as no surprise now. The moment I decided to pursue residency, I was all in for the two-year residency program stretch. But when that time came, there was something holding me back. I found myself interested in other areas beyond critical care (my original PGY2 interest). My co-residents already had their itineraries mapped out and application materials in before I could even read the program descriptions. I remember standing in a circle with our director during ASHP's Midyear Clinical Meeting networking among pharmacy leaders. I lost track of how many times I had to divert the conversation before it was my turn to comment "I'm not really sure I want to pursue a PGY2 program" when asked about what specialty I chose. At this point in your career, you're surrounded by so many eager and driven individuals that my uncertainty made me feel as though I was "giving up." That was my biggest struggle. It was after that conference that I realized I wasn't giving up, but simply wasn't more passionate about one specialty over another. There is an enormous value in a second year, and I would absolutely encourage anyone considering a specialty to go all in. But for those of you who haven't decided what specialty that is, don't be afraid to start your job search but with the mindset of working just as hard in your first year of practice as you would in a second year residency. *Make it a habit early on to challenge yourself, and you will be successful.*

DETERMINING YOUR CARE PRACTICE AREA(S)—SAY "YES"

Following my residency completion, I applied for a job at the same hospital. Believe it or not, this was a no brainer. For me, there was a greater value in staying at the same institution to practice in a familiar environment where I could focus on being a patient care practitioner and contribute to a multidisciplinary team. I felt as though I could put more energy into developing relationships and starting my true career.

Soon into my practice, we were short on staff in the emergency department, so I started working weekend shifts there. The antimicrobial stewardship program was in transition between new coordinators so I, along with another pharmacist, stepped into that role. When I was in pharmacy school, the infectious disease (ID) course might as well have been taught in Spanish. I'm sure the expression on my face was comical. For that reason, I was eager to postpone my residency ID rotation at all costs but realizing there was no way to avoid it, I put in the work. I spent many late nights at the hospital, and it finally paid off. A few months later in a new career position, I was given the opportunity to bridge the transition period between the previous and incoming ID pharmacy coordinators. Never in a million years would I have expected to jump at the opportunity to take on this role, and now it's the first thing I look at when I chart review.

We tend to shy away from the areas we aren't as confident in or tasks that are unfamiliar. Recognize the questions that come up often and be the person who is curious enough to find the answers than the one who asks the questions. Identify your own weaknesses and conquer them so when challenges arise you're not caught off guard.

KNOWING WHAT I KNOW NOW

I am grateful for the road bumps and detours that led me to my current position. I ended up choosing not to be a clinical pharmacy specialist but a clinical pharmacy generalist specializing in a multitude of areas including nutrition, internal medicine, surgery, and emergency medicine.

My life plan didn't fall into place for me from the start. I racked up some extra graduate credits and tried my hand at a different profession, but was lucky to find a job I love in the end. No matter what field you choose, at some point, I'm willing to bet almost every single person has thought about a new career direction. For me, it was before my career even began.

Fortunately, in this profession, your opportunities are endless. For some of you, climbing the career ladder will fulfill your professional goals; for others, it's the patient interventions. All of your paths will be different, and your interests will evolve with your career. I cannot speak from years of experience on the job, but I can look back at the last years in college, graduate school, pharmacy school, and residency and say with certainty that it was completely worth it.

Whether you live to work or work to live, these next few years are so important for setting the foundation of your career. *Step out of your comfort zone, learn at least one new thing every day, and continue to investigate your options until your career is right for you.*

All the best,

Kelley

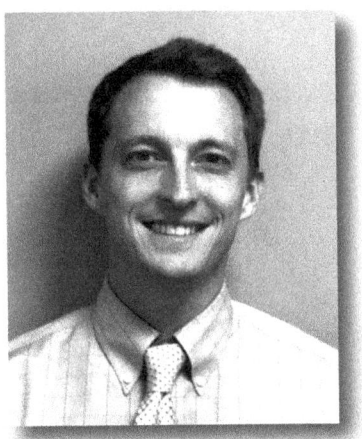

Jeffrey (Jeff) Millard
PharmD, MBA, BCPS

Keeping the End in Mind

Jeff is a dedicated pharmacist and a dynamic leader. He is thoughtful and detail oriented, and can develop processes and influence people across the spectrum of health system to create positive change. His focus is to provide his patients the best possible care at the most appropriate cost.

Jeff is currently Ambulatory Pharmacy Operations Coordinator, Banner Health, Phoenix, Arizona. He previously completed a postgraduate year 1 (PGY1)/PGY2 health-system pharmacy administration residency at Banner Health. Jeff earned his PharmD degree and MBA at Idaho State University, Meridian.

Jeff's advice is: **Weigh the pros and the cons. Choosing residency is not an easy decision, but worth the time necessary to study the many options. I wish you the best of luck as you consider your "end in mind"—wherever that may take you!**

Dear Pharmacy Colleague,

I have always been a fan of the book *The 7 Habits of Highly Effective People*, in which the author describes seven habits that, if developed, will lead you to be a more effective person. My favorite habit encourages readers to have an "end in mind." This means envisioning in your mind what you can't see with your eyes. It would include questions such as *Who do you want to be? What do you want to become? What do you want to accomplish during your life?* Focusing on my end in mind, including what I pictured myself doing throughout my career, was a central part of my decision to pursue a pharmacy residency.

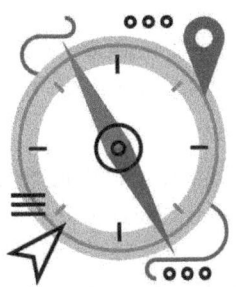

My path to becoming a pharmacist started in 10th grade, with the encouragement of my biology teacher whose wife was a pharmacist. My friends and I enjoyed our association with this particular teacher, so we would always arrive to class a few minutes early. Our conversations would regularly turn to how much enjoyment and satisfaction his wife received from her work as a pharmacist. Eventually, after job shadowing, researching, and visiting my state's college of pharmacy, I decided that pharmacy was the career for me.

If you fast forward seven years and countless nightmares about organic chemistry exams and carbon bonds, you would find me sitting in orientation as a P1 pharmacy student at Idaho State University College of Pharmacy. At the same time as we were embarking on intense didactic coursework and studying, I started to learn about the opportunities and career options afforded to pharmacists including residency training. Finding these new avenues and opportunities was fascinating; I became proactive in meeting with different people and groups to learn more. As I interviewed different types of pharmacists and asked about their jobs and their likes and dislikes, I started to develop my career vision.

DECISION TIME

At the start of P4 year, it was time for me to start making decisions. Did I want to pursue a residency? The clinical concepts and knowledge about medications I gained in pharmacy school fascinated me. Cardiology was the topic I enjoyed most. I couldn't wait to start rotations and help real patients. At the same time, I also found myself intrigued by the business and administration side of pharmacy, gaining exposure through my Master's in Business Administration (MBA) program. I tried to figure out how I could get the best of both worlds—pharmacy and business. Through a classmate, I learned about health-system pharmacy administration (HSPA) residencies. This seemed to be the answer I had been searching for! I knew that a general PGY1 year would help solidify the clinical concepts I learned in school and believed the addition of a pharmacy administration-focused PGY2 would set me up for the career to which I aspired.

Various other considerations also played into my decision to pursue residency training:

1. **Encouragement from a young age to obtain as much education and training as possible.** It is a competitive world full of competitive people. Worthwhile training and education will help set you apart.

2. **1:1 time with preceptors.** Being able to stand shoulder to shoulder with experts in different fields of pharmacy is a unique opportunity of residency. As a resident, you are able to ask questions, learn from different preceptors while observing their practice style, and get a snapshot of what pharmacy

practice is like in various specialties. Compared to being observers as P4 pharmacy students, pharmacy residents are an integral part of the patient care team. They are consulted to provide correct answers regarding complex medication management questions involving multiple overlapping disease states. Preceptors help residents develop and hone problem-solving skills that allow efficient and effective management of even the most critically ill patients.

3. **Flexibility.** I wasn't ready to decide at the end of pharmacy school exactly what job I wanted to do for the next 40 years. I wanted to explore many options. I knew residency would allow me to do that. Although required rotations and experiences are associated with every residency program, there is a high level of flexibility too. Residents are able to request more exposure to areas they are interested in.

4. **Residency is kind of a really long job interview.** I always felt that a one-hour job interview was insufficient for an employer to determine if an employee will fit in with a company, and for a candidate to decide if he or she will fit in with that company. Residency is a 3000+ hour job interview, and that's only after the first year. By the end of a successfully completed residency, you will probably have the chance to either stay on where you trained or—because pharmacy is a small world where everyone knows everyone—you will be able to use your newly developed network and colleagues to find your preferred position.

5. **Variety of career opportunities.** The same job opportunities that were available before residency were still open to me after completing residency. However, I was pleasantly surprised at the new opportunities that started to appear as my residency ended. There were people from different companies I had met during residency who tried recruiting me to work for them. There were also administrative pharmacy positions open across the country that required completion of a pharmacy residency to even apply. Without residency, I would not have been able to consider these other opportunities.

Having just completed my HSPA residency, I have spent time reflecting on the past two years and the growth I have seen in myself.

A FEW TAKEAWAYS FROM MY RESIDENCY EXPERIENCES

The essential role a pharmacist plays on the patient care team. The need for a medication expert to carefully examine each patient's drug therapies was frequently evident. It was not uncommon in our hospital to see patient medication lists exceeding 20 different medications. Each member of the patient care team has an area of expertise—physicians are experts at diagnosing, nurses provide continuous support and serve as the liaison between the patient and the medical team, and dietitians ensure patients are getting the proper nutrition during their hospital stay. Pharmacists complete the team with their training and ability to tailor medication regimens to each patient.

The importance of regular reflection time. Pharmacy residencies specifically require learners to take time and evaluate their performance during each rotation. The reflection process includes examining what went well, and more importantly, what did not go well. Goals are set, and plans made for how specific weaknesses can be overcome during the next rotation. This was often a very uncomfortable process. Talking about your weaknesses is no one's favorite pastime, and I was no different. One of my biggest weaknesses identified early during residency was my fear of being wrong. For example, during the early parts of residency, if a question came up on patient care rounds I did not completely know the answer to, I was always quick to suggest I would research the question and return and report my recommendation to the team. Although this strategy is not fundamentally wrong, it is important to give accurate and evidence-based answers to clinical questions my preceptors identified. They encouraged me, when appropriate, to attempt to talk through the question and answer. From then on, when faced with a difficult question during rounds that I wasn't completely sure of, I would start by succinctly explaining what I did know about the topic. I would then ask additional questions. More times than not, these two strategies stimulated discussion among the other providers that led us to an agreeable and successful medication management strategy. This approach helped me become more confident at answering difficult questions on the spot. Identifying that weakness and fixing it made me a more effective pharmacist.

Through this and other examples, I quickly came to realize the value of regular reflection time to consider feedback and progress toward my goals. I have seen the value of continuing this reflection process in my short time being out of residency. In my current work position, I have short- and long-term goals. Reflecting on a daily basis about how the day went, taking time weekly and monthly to examine progress toward my goals, and making course corrections as necessary enables me to be more efficient and laser-focused on the most important tasks I need to complete to see success.

The results of residency training are really in the hands of the residents. If residents come every day determined to learn and be engaged, they will accomplish great things. If residents are passive and wait for great opportunities to find them, they will likely miss many chances. As opportunities arose for me, I learned the benefits of volunteering for projects. This was especially true because I sought to be involved with projects that had unfamiliar topics. My second year longitudinal administration research project involved standardizing workflows in ambulatory infusion centers. I am almost positive they didn't teach us how to do this in pharmacy school! During the project, I carried out gap analyses, implemented new workflows, and asked thousands of questions. This project took me out of my comfort zone. There were a lot of barriers that worked to hinder our progress including employees' resistance to change, conflicting opinions about workflows, and technological limitations. However, tenacity and grit allowed us to push past those barriers and achieve success. Little did I know that this residency project would turn into a large part of the role I would assume upon completing residency!

Deciding whether or not to pursue a residency is a question every pharmacy student will likely spend time considering. For me, the decision was made much easier when I thought about where I wanted to end up in my career. After deciding to pursue residency, I was lucky to match at a great program led by highly qualified pharmacy leaders. To add to my good fortune, the same company hired me after residency to fill a position that matches my interests and skillset. Even better, I work with a highly talented and motivated team that pushes me to be better every single day. Pursuing residency training was the right decision for me.

As you compare and examine your career options, I would encourage you to take time and put thought into what career path you will be most passionate about. *Weigh the pros and the cons. It is not an easy decision but worth taking the time needed to examine the many options.*

Thank you for reading this letter. I wish you the best of luck as you consider your "end in mind"—wherever that may take you!

Jeff

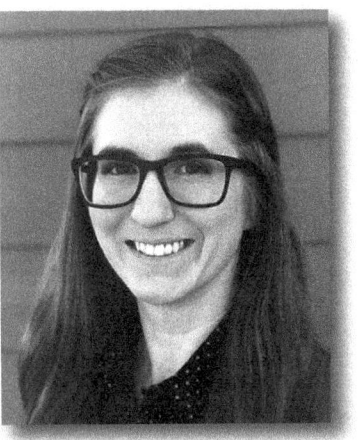

Whitney Mortensen
PharmD, MBA, BCPS

Taking the Path Less Traveled

Whitney exhibits many characteristics you would expect of a high performer, including dedication, efficiency, and intelligence. What makes Whitney stand out is her open mind, ability to get people on her side, and keen insight in most situations. Whitney's ability to grow and improve is amazing. She has a unique way of learning from any situation and then using that experience to keep improving. With Whitney, each day is literally better than the last.

Whitney is currently a drug information specialist at Intermountain Healthcare in Taylorsville, Utah. She completed her accredited postgraduate year (PGY) 2 health-system pharmacy administration residency and her accredited PGY1 pharmacy residency at Intermountain Healthcare located in Murray, Utah. Whitney earned her PharmD degree from Roseman University of Health Sciences, College of Pharmacy, and her MBA from Roseman University of Health Sciences, College of Business, both located in South Jordan, Utah.

Whitney's advice is: **Make decisions about your career based not on what you feel you should do but what you truly want to do. In my opinion, that is the best way to build a fulfilling and meaningful career.**

Dear Pharmacy Colleague,

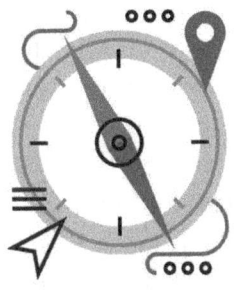

As with many pharmacy students, I was uncertain which area of pharmacy would be the best fit for me. To make a more educated decision about my career path, I tried to gain an understanding of pharmacy practice in a variety of areas. I considered all sorts of possible options ranging from ownership of an independent community pharmacy to clinical veterinary pharmacy. My career interests had always been diverse, so I wanted to gain experiences in different settings and specialties. I remember explaining to many preceptors and mentors that I liked to dabble in different areas of practice but had not found a specialty I was truly passionate about. I spent some time working as an intern at a community pharmacy chain but realized that that was not the best fit for me. I knew it would be essential for me to keep my options open. I also knew obtaining additional clinical training would be key. It was a gradual process that led me to decide postgraduate training (residency training) was my best option. It would allow me to investigate various clinical areas and to make an informed decision about my future. After making this decision, I still found myself at an impasse. I pondered: *What type of residency program would provide me with the most growth opportunities and job prospects as a new pharmacist?*

I enjoyed many of the advanced pharmacy practice experiences (APPEs) I had as a student, but at the end of the rotation I was always more than ready to move on to something new. I applied to residency programs that would allow me to gain experience in various clinical areas caring for both adult and pediatric patients. I also applied to some health-system pharmacy administration programs. I was working on a Master of Business Administration degree concurrently with a Doctor of Pharmacy degree and had always known at some point I would want to move into a formal leadership position. The decision to apply to different types of residency programs was driven by my desire to have a broad understanding of many different pharmacy settings. I received all that and more when I matched with the two-year health-system pharmacy administration residency program at Intermountain Healthcare. Completing a residency is beneficial in terms of developing and expanding your skills as a clinician. This clinical knowledge, while its importance cannot be overstated, is not the most crucial thing I gained from residency training.

IMPORTANT SKILLS THAT TRANSLATED DIRECTLY TO PROFESSIONAL ROLES

The most important skills I learned in residency now help me to effectively work and function in a professional setting. Balancing responsibilities on rotation with longitudinal projects and tasks pushed me to improve my time and project management skills, as well as my ability to work efficiently. An essential skill was learning to appropriately prioritize work with multiple preceptors from different rotations. Another part of this was learning to say "no." Residency was the first time in my life where I was presented with more opportunities than I could pursue. I had to think carefully about when to take on additional assignments so I would not neglect my other responsibilities. At first, it was difficult to adjust my way of thinking to achieve this, but it was essential so I could consistently produce high-quality work.

Residency taught me how to work autonomously. If I had identified barriers or needed clarification on the expectations or scope of a project or presentation, the onus was on me to seek out additional information and ask questions. Working through many of these situations, I learned to critically think about the topic and brainstorm possible solutions. This skill is invaluable. In residency, knowing how to effectively communicate with others both orally and in writing was imperative. With these skills, practice is the best way to hone your abilities. Residency presents frequent opportunities to practice and improve these skills via formal and informal presentations and written projects. My residency training allowed me to develop my abilities to communicate clearly in both clinical and nonclinical settings. I learned how to pass along information about a patient's status to another pharmacist, how to compose a concise e-mail to request project feedback from stakeholders, how to approach physicians to recommend a change in therapy, and how to express myself during meetings. Essentially, I gained real experience as a professional, and I continue to make use of and build on that knowledge. The biggest lesson of my residency training, though, came when I had to make a decision about my future career trajectory.

OPTIONS AND DECISIONS

Near the end of my second year of residency, I was fortunate to have options in the form of two very different choices for my first post-residency job as a pharmacist—inpatient pharmacy manager at the adult flagship hospital in the health system where I completed my residency training, or drug information specialist at the corporate office in the same health system. As a resident, I had months of experience with the teams from each position. That, however, was one of the only similarities between my job opportunities.

Option 1: Inpatient Pharmacy Manager. In this situation, the inpatient pharmacy manager had task-based responsibilities and worked mainly with pharmacists, pharmacy technicians, and pharmacy interns. There were certainly aspects of this position that appealed to me. I knew many of the people I would be working with as I had completed my first year of residency at that hospital. I always planned to take on a formal leadership role at some point in my career; as a manager with direct reports, I would have the opportunity to lead both pharmacists and technicians. Working with my colleagues, I could implement continuous quality improvement projects to better the existing processes and improve medication and patient safety. I would be able to apply the business concepts I learned as a student to real-world situations.

Option 2: Drug Information Specialist. A drug information specialist in this health system had project-based responsibilities and worked with pharmacists and other healthcare professionals from many different backgrounds. There were many facets of this position that I found desirable. I had a few rotations with the drug information team and others working in medication-use policy; in fact, the experiences I had related to these areas were the only ones that I did not want to leave when the rotation ended. I enjoyed the work, particularly because the projects I completed could potentially have a positive impact on the lives of thousands of patients throughout the health system. Additionally, the position would offer a significant amount of clinical variety, as well as many opportunities for involvement and participation in committees. Experience in drug information would also allow me to continue developing skills that are desirable and easily transferrable to any position, especially verbal and written communication.

On paper, working as an inpatient pharmacy manager may have been the logical next step for a health-system pharmacy administration resident with a business degree. It was arguably the path that many colleagues expected me to take. It would have provided me with many great chances to grow and learn, particularly in my knowledge of operations. It was, however, not the best choice for me. I still hope to work in a formal leadership position in the future; however, I felt that I needed time to practice independently first. This was in part to ensure that I could continue assessing my own performance, expanding my knowledge, and developing my skillset of my own accord. Also, a healthy work–life balance is exceptionally important to me and, as my residency program director emphasized, you have to create that balance for yourself; no one else will do it for you. It is especially challenging to break the habit of working long days and weekends, but having a more flexible schedule certainly makes it easier to find that balance.

It has been nearly two years since I started my first post-residency job, and I do not regret choosing to begin my career as a drug information specialist. At the end of the day, the biggest lesson I learned from my residency training is that there is no set path you have to follow professionally or personally, so do what you think will be best for you as an individual.

I hope that you will not make decisions about your career based on what you feel you *should* do but, rather, what you truly *want* to do. In my opinion, that is the best way to build a fulfilling and meaningful career.

I encourage you to be thoughtful about the decisions you make that impact your future, and I wish you the best of luck as you begin your career as a pharmacist.

Kind regards,

Whitney

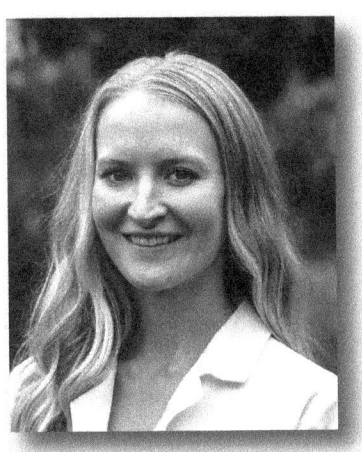

Ryan P. Nottingham
PharmD

Go Out There and Play Hard; Then Look to Your Future

Ryan exudes professionalism, applies an appropriate filter, listens attentively, and recommends improvements that are carefully thought out for the success of her team. She strives for excellence, while quietly but confidently raising the bar, and has a passion for circling back and aligning her focus around the patient or colleague. Ryan demonstrates great compassion in her natural draw toward patients dealing with catastrophic illness. She designed pharmacy services in palliative care as a student and resident.

Ryan is currently a Clinical Pharmacist, Lifebridge Health Northwest Hospital, Randallstown, Maryland. She completed her accredited postgraduate year 1 (PGY1) pharmacy residency at Providence St. Peter Hospital, Olympia, Washington and received her PharmD degree from Washington State University, Spokane.

Ryan's advice is: **Surround yourself with people who not only support your dreams but also help you realize bigger and better dreams and push you to reach them.**

Dear Pharmacy Colleague,

To begin, you will notice that my husband Jimmy pops up a lot in this letter. It happens

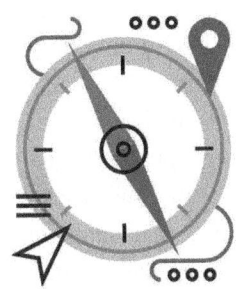

because he has been my pre-pharmacy school classmate, coworker, pharmacy school classmate, co-resident, and best friend. When I say that he has been with me every step of the way, it is not an exaggeration. *My best piece of advice is to surround yourself with people who not only support your dreams but also help you realize bigger and better dreams and push you to reach them.* If you can convince one of them to stick with you for life, it's even better.

Two days after our wedding, Jimmy and I started our residency together at a community hospital in Olympia, Washington. It was not exactly how we expected to spend our honeymoon, but it makes for a good laugh. We ate, slept, and breathed pharmacy that year. It was what we talked about every morning and every night when getting ready for bed. That is, if we were lucky enough to see each other at all that day. There was one rotation where he would get to work at 6:30 in the morning. That same rotation cycle, I started work at 3:00 p.m. He would stop by my service line to say good night before leaving because it was the only time we would see each other that day. Residency is hard. It is physically, mentally, and emotionally exhausting. But I would not trade those 12 months for anything.

I chose residency because I wanted to be a proactive pharmacist. When looking at my different career options, pharmacists seemed to come to the table *after* decisions were made. I wanted to be there to help *make* the decisions. As a drug information expert, I wanted to speak up at the time when therapy options were considered. Working in a hospital or clinic was my best opportunity to have this career, and the best way to get there was through residency. Pharmacy school lays the groundwork for a career in hospital pharmacy. I was a confident student, ready to take on any challenges life and career would throw at me. Looking back, I would not have been ready to work in a hospital directly out of school. I could not have done the work justice. I could not have joined the clinical dialogue required of a hospital pharmacist. Residency provides vocabulary, context, and knowledge depth that simply cannot be shoehorned into three or four years of pharmacy school.

As much as I loved my program and believe that everyone should consider it as an option, I recognize that residency is not for everyone. It is a year of saying *yes* to a lot of people, except you. You will need to rearrange your life to accommodate others. You will bring work home. People will constantly question your knowledge, and sometimes it will not be in a positive way. Every time you get to feel confident in the work you do, you will be shifted into a new service line. If you can make it past that, the knowledge learned and the relationships formed make it worthwhile. The most important relationships you can gain will be with your residency director, preceptors, co-residents, and students.

Find a residency director who will be on your side because, to be honest, not everyone will be. This will be uncomfortable for you. But, if you have a director who supports you, you will get through it. There will be preceptors who will look at you like a chore, and administrators who will look at you like chattel. Further, figure out who the true educators are in your group of preceptors. Not all preceptors are created equal. Find the people who are excited about their job, always learning, and genuinely interested in helping you achieve your goals. Listen to them and take their information to heart. People are more likely to teach to active learners. Be a friend to your co-residents because they are among the few people who understand what you are going through. Do not let others speak poorly of your co-residents. This is not a competition. You are all there to learn—and trust me—you will. Work with student pharmacists. The very best way to learn is through teaching. Complete your teaching certificate. It is not something you will likely go back to do at a later date. Working with students keeps your mind fresh as they ask questions to which you know the answers as well as questions you had not thought of yet.

Our PGY1 was an amazing experience. Our program gave us the confidence to apply to PGY2 and fellowship programs. I applied to six programs and received six interviews. On a scale of one to 10, I felt I had good odds. One program, in particular, seemed to have stolen the blueprint to my dream career. During my interview, I felt an instant connection with the pharmacist preceptors. The director and I met prior to the interview at a conference and hit it off. We did a phone interview and texted; she even helped coordinate interview times with Jimmy's program. This was a team that I felt I was already a part of. It felt like the position was mine. When Match Day game, Jimmy had his position; I did not. Trials and tribulations are the teachers, my friend. I hear it builds character. Although my PGY2 experience was short, to say the least, I would not change it. I applied to fantastic programs, in beautiful areas, filled with amazing pharmacists. Practice makes perfect, and it holds true for interviewing. Never take any interview for granted as it either leads to a new career or insight on how you can improve your interviewing skills. *Rejection hurts, but it is something you need to let go. Learn what you can from the experience and then look to the future.*

Do not let a single setback dictate your abilities and future possibilities. There are certifications and specialty traineeships all across the country that allow you to improve your knowledge base in whatever field interests you. As I said before, residency is not for everyone. However, allowing yourself to fall short of your dreams is not acceptable. No one takes organic chemistry because it is fun. No one studies sunup to sundown because it is easy. These are all stepping stones to reach our goals. *If you are not where you want to be, keep moving. Knowledge never goes out of style.*

Jimmy's program had us move from Washington State to Maryland. We left behind all of our family, friends, and our entire pharmacy network. I started from scratch when applying for hospital positions. I did not have any friends of friends or old classmates to help me in my new town. I was also applying to positions at the most difficult time of the year—right after residency and pharmacy school graduations. Luckily, residency is a language that is spoken across the country. I received my job offer one month after arriving in Maryland. If I had chosen to forgo residency, if I had taken a hospital position directly out of school, I do not think I would have found employment so quickly.

A quote that has played a significant role in my life comes from a short story by Toshio Mori entitled *The Woman Who Makes Swell Doughnuts*:

"...play, play hard, go out there and play hard. You will be glad later for everything you have done with all your might."

In this moment, an elderly woman is discussing her grandchildren playing in the backyard. You get a sense of the longing in this character, how she reminisces about times where she was able to work and play. Although she seems happy in her present situation, it still stirred in me this idea of putting my strength into each action, whether it is work, life, or play. I do not want to look back in my golden years and regret. I do not want to regret missed opportunities, inaction, or always taking the easy way. We can forgive so many grievances; stagnation is not one of them. I also love that I still think back to this quote, which I read for English class in high school. Walking into class that day, I did not know that the story would strike me as it did.

We seldom realize the most important things in our lives the moment they happen. You never know when a stranger will become your best friend, or start a hobby that will become a passion, or take a job that will become a calling. I certainly did not recognize that the smug guy with the mohawk in my biomedical ethics class would end up being my husband. Take each day, recognizing and respecting the sheer power in each moment.

Now, go out there and play hard.

Warmly,

Ryan

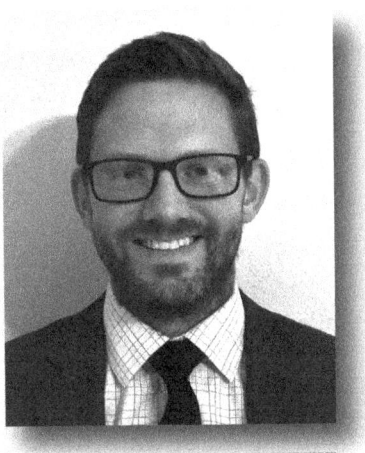

Jeremy D. Price
PharmD

Every Day of Residency Is a Unique Learning Opportunity

Jeremy began his professional journey at Riverside University Health System as a postgraduate year 1 (PGY1) resident pharmacist with interests in acute care, critical care, and emergency medicine. As part of the inaugural class of residents, he was instrumental in providing information for ASHP accreditation surveyors for the newly accredited residency and also provided feedback for the overall improvement of the residency program.

Jeremy has shown tremendous growth as a pharmacist and a person. His involvement with quality improvement projects and provider education has contributed to improved drug therapy management. Jeremy has formed strong relationships with healthcare staff of various disciplines and has become a trustworthy and reliable member of the healthcare team. His personable manner and steadfast work ethic has earned him the respect of his colleagues throughout his training and as a staff member.

Jeremy is currently a Clinical Pharmacist at Riverside University Health System. He completed his PGY1 residency at Riverside University Health System, Riverside, California and received his PharmD degree at the University of Iowa, College of Pharmacy, Iowa City and his BS in Biology at San Diego State University, California.

Jeremy's advice is: **If you are not 100% certain about what you want to do after graduation, you are not alone. Simply weigh the risks and benefits, and if the benefits of residency outweigh the risks, then go for it!**

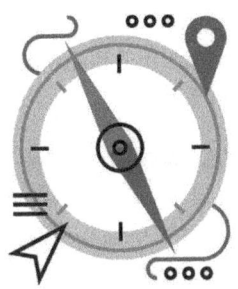

Dear Pharmacy Colleague,

Whether you are in your first year of pharmacy school or your last, you have at some point either thought about or been asked about residency. For many of you, the choice to pursue residency after graduation is clear. For others, it is hazy at best.

It can be an agonizing decision with many factors to consider: *What are your short- and long-term goals? What kind of position(s) are you interested in? Are you interested in a particular specialty? What type of facility? Is location important?* If you are still weighing your options, perhaps you would be interested in hearing about my experience before, during, and after residency.

For me, residency was a foregone conclusion. I have always been interested in acute care pharmacy and the thought of having a year or two to practice as a licensed pharmacist, under the watchful eyes of experienced preceptors, was very appealing. I also did not want to have any regrets should I opt out of residency and find that the opportunities I thought would be available to me were, in fact, not. Unfortunately, the job market is not as favorable for new graduates as it once was and setting yourself apart is more important than ever. Now, residency does not guarantee you your dream job, or any job for that matter, but it does make you a more attractive prospect in a very competitive market. Even if the jobs you are interested in do not currently require residency training, that may not always be the case. In fact, both ASHP and the American College of Clinical Pharmacy (ACCP) have suggested that by 2020, residency training or equivalent experience should be a prerequisite for all pharmacists in direct patient care roles. In any case, I can assure you there are many good reasons to consider residency.

OPPORTUNITY

Residency gives you the opportunity to apply what you learned in pharmacy school, expand your base of knowledge, and gain experience in various settings with diverse patient populations. You also have the opportunity to improve your problem-solving skills, develop your communication skills, and become a stronger leader and a more mature, confident pharmacist. You will become more familiar with drug therapy management and the drugs, doses, routes, frequencies, and durations involved. You may be involved in and learn to work under the stress of a code situation or navigate the complicated health insurance system. I still remember the first code I responded to. I was so nervous—my heart was pounding. I had a hard time finding the medications, and then I fumbled with them once I found them. I had trouble remembering doses and timing of administration. Luckily, one of my preceptors was there to help me. Since then I have responded to many codes. I still fumble with medication from time to time, but my heart doesn't beat quite as fast, and I am much more confident thanks to my preceptors and the experience I gained during residency.

TIME MANAGEMENT, COMMUNICATION SKILLS, AND WORKING WITH TEAMS

Being a successful resident requires excellent time management, communication skills, and the ability to work effectively as a team member. You will be involved in various projects, asked to do several lectures, participate in journal clubs, compose newsletters, conduct research, and precept for rotating students. This will require you to manage your time wisely and stay in constant contact with your preceptors, project advisor, and program director. Your research project will require weeks of your time; may involve several people; require you to harness resources; and seek help, advice, and guidance. Make sure you keep interested parties in the loop about what is going on with particular projects and with your residency in general. I have always taken pride in my communication skills, but during residency I realized that while I was good at communicating one-on-one, I was not as good at communicating with larger groups of people via emailing, etc. It is something I continue to work on, but experiences in residency enabled me to make significant improvements in that area.

Every day of residency is a unique learning opportunity. Embrace it. Take everything you can from each experience. It can get pretty hectic and stressful at times, so make sure you take some time for yourself outside of residency. Try to establish a comfortable work–life balance. There will also be times when you will feel inadequate, even stupid. I know I did. It can be frustrating, but this is one aspect of residency that makes it so wonderful. You are not expected to know everything as a resident. However, you are expected to learn, develop your areas of weakness, and take initiative to better yourself. In residency, you can make mistakes. Just remember, you have a life-line—your preceptor. Out of residency, you will be working without a net, so to speak. So, take on challenges that you might otherwise avoid. Sign up for rotations in areas of weakness. For me, that was oncology. So, I selected Hematology–Oncology as one of my two elective rotations, and I can tell you I am much better for it. Take advantage of opportunities to work with preceptors and pharmacy colleagues, medical residents, and attending physicians. There is so much you can learn from one another. During residency, I formed wonderful relationships with pharmacists and physicians, many of whom I still work with. Working together is easier because of an established level of confidence, trust, and respect.

THE RIGHT FIT

Where you do your training is nearly as important as doing residency at all. Luckily, the number and variety of available residency positions is greater than it has ever been. Whether you are interested in acute care, ambulatory, community, or managed care pharmacy, there is a residency for you. Look for a residency that fits your interests and personality. You can gather much of the basic information about a program online or in brochures, but many programs look very similar on paper. Gather as much information as you can in person, on the phone, or via email. Go to the ASHP Midyear Clinical Meeting (MCM) and talk to the current residents; try to get a feel for the program. Attending the MCM during both my third and fourth year of pharmacy school was a wonderful opportunity to meet like-minded people and learn about the residency programs. If it is convenient, you should consider visiting the facility and learn as much as you can during your interview(s). Remember, you are interviewing the residency as much as the residency is interviewing you. Consider programs that are flexible in terms of your interests and forming your rotation schedule. Look for programs with a variety of possible elective rotations. Explore a residency in a particular facility or geographic area that you might be interested in after residency. You never know when a residency could lead to a job.

Ultimately, I selected my residency based on a number of factors, not the least of which were the positive interactions I had with pharmacists and staff during fourth year rotations, the complexity of the patient population and associated learning opportunities, the flexibility of the program, and the location. I made the right choice. I had a wonderful residency experience and now work at the facility where I did my training.

GET INVOLVED

If you are an underclassman and you are considering residency, I encourage you to start building a strong residency application. Get involved in activities that show your interest in the profession, advance the profession, and/or help the community. Look for a pharmacy job while you are in school. You don't have to work a ton of hours, but some experience helps. Participate in events that help you develop your skills— patient communication, immunization, blood pressure monitoring, finger sticks for blood glucose, etc. Take on a leadership position and attend pharmacy organization meetings. Network and learn about the profession. During pharmacy school I participated in mobile community clinics and flu shot drives, volunteered with Habitat for Humanity, worked as an intern pharmacist at the Veterans Affairs hospital, presented a poster at MCM, was a committee member for my pharmacy school's Information Technology Committee, and was the Vice President of Policy for the University of Iowa chapter of ASHP. I was also a member of local and national pharmacy associations. Even if you decide to forgo residency, the knowledge and experience you gain and the connections you make participating in these activities will be beneficial as you seek employment and begin your career.

OPPORTUNITIES AFTER RESIDENCY

After residency, there are many avenues of pharmacy to explore including a PGY2, board certification, or adjunct faculty at a local pharmacy school. When I completed my residency, I was offered a position as a clinical pharmacist at the hospital where I did my residency training. I decided not to pursue a PGY2 residency, partially because I did not find one particular area of acute care pharmacy that I had enough interest in to justify a second year of residency. I am now lucky enough to work in areas throughout the hospital—inpatient pharmacy, intravenous therapy room, medical/surgical units, intensive care units, progressive care units, and emergency department. I really enjoy the variety and opportunity to gain the knowledge and experience each unit has to offer. I can honestly say I learn something new every day.

Looking back, I do not regret one minute of my residency. I made a few mistakes, and I learned from them. I had a great deal of success and formed wonderful relationships. Most importantly, I grew. I am more mature, knowledgeable, and confident. There is still a lot I don't know, but I am more motivated than ever to be better at my job, for myself and for my patients. In the end, residency training gave me the ability to provide safer, more effective pharmaceutical care and the opportunity to practice at the top of my license. I will forever be grateful to the preceptors, mentors, and even pharmacy students who helped me along the way.

If you are not 100% certain about what you want to do after graduation, you are not alone. Simply weigh the risks and benefits, and if the benefits of residency outweigh the risks, then go for it!

Jeremy

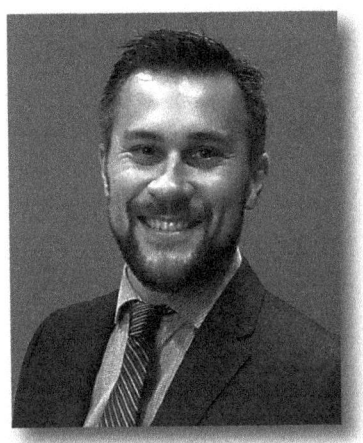

Joshua N. Raub
PharmD, BCPS

Setting High Goals and Continuous Self-Reflection Leads to Success

Josh credits his early career success to a principle of continually raising the bar for himself. He ascribes three action steps to sustaining his achievements and provides wisdom to recent pharmacy graduates who wish to hit the ground running with their new career.

Josh is currently a Clinical Pharmacist Specialist in internal medicine at Detroit Receiving Hospital and Assistant Residency Program Director for the postgraduate year 1 (PGY1) pharmacy residency program at the Detroit Medical Center. Josh holds adjunct faculty positions at the Wayne State University School of Medicine and College of Pharmacy. He has served on the ASHP Section Advisory Group for Preceptor Skills Development. Josh has received numerous awards for precepting from Wayne State University, in addition to ASHP Foundation's 2016 New Preceptor of the Year. Josh received his PharmD degree from the Eugene Applebaum College of Pharmacy and Health Sciences at Wayne State University and completed a PGY1 pharmacy residency at The Johns Hopkins Hospital in Baltimore, Maryland.

Josh's advice is: **Continue to raise the bar for yourself. Progress is never stationary, and the same should be true of your goals!**

Dear Pharmacy Colleague,

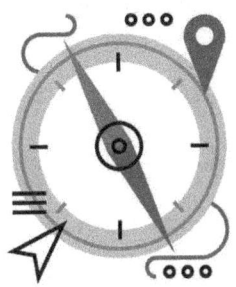

The wondrous beauty of hindsight is that it is 20/20. The ability to dissect the past and identify steps that led to both success and failure is an amazing tool to apply to your future goals. I have always considered self-reflection to be one of the greatest aspects of future success. As pharmacists, the process is innate to us. We are often involved in research, whether it is designing a study, participating in one, or evaluating results; we continually posit hypotheses and reflect on their outcomes.

The same thing can be said of our work ethic and desire for success. We continually conduct post-hoc analyses of our day-to-day workings and then take prior knowledge of our mistakes and accomplishments and mold them into a new process with the goal of improvement. Like clinical research, success cannot always be found and we may not always meet our desired outcome, but valuable lessons will always be gained to move forward. Growing up, I was often told, *"You'll have no idea of knowing where you are going if you don't stop, take a moment, and look where you came from."*

It has been a few years since I graduated from pharmacy school. Similar to most graduates, I was proud of what I had accomplished, and a sense of invincibility grew inside of me. This ambitious pride, however, was soon tempered with vulnerability because the path ahead of me was largely unknown. After completing my pharmacy degree with a predetermined curriculum to follow, it was the first time in my life that I was unaware of what to expect next. My future and subsequent career was a *tabula rasa*—a blank slate.

Hindsight, as I mentioned earlier, provides a crystal-clear vision of the past. Although I have only practiced as a licensed pharmacist for awhile, I believe the first few years after graduation are the most important to propel your career. As a new pharmacist, the possibilities are endless as to where you want to establish your niche in our profession. You possess an armamentarium of specialized knowledge that truly sets you apart from your peers and an eagerness to improve patient care. However, like any skilled professional, it is crucial to possess the right tools to master the trade. When I reflect on my journey from pharmacy school to residency to my current position, I have maintained a consistent work philosophy that has been beneficial to helping me achieve my goals. The objective that I aim for every day is to continually raise the bar for myself. I have found this to be motivating, but also frustrating at times. The tricky part of this philosophy is to not set the bar to an unreachable height. *I have discovered the act of "raising the bar" is a constant dance between exceeding your expectations while avoiding your breaking point.* Nevertheless, it fuels your inner drive and motivation, steering your pursuit for success.

As you embark on your career, I want to provide sage wisdom on maximizing your potential, and provide tools to apply to your innate pursuit of success. Through trial and error, **I have discovered three main action steps to help achieve the raise-the-bar mentality:**

- Identify and utilize a mentor
- Embody the underdog mantra
- Seek out challenges

BENEFITING FROM THE MENTOR-MENTEE RELATIONSHIP

During my fourth year of pharmacy school, I was still contemplating residency and whether I should pursue it. I was aware of the challenges that residency entailed, and I was certain that I wanted to be a preceptor in the future. Therefore, I focused on residency programs that aligned with my goals and interests. I was eager to develop my teaching and precepting skills so I sought out programs that were affiliated with colleges of pharmacy, offered teaching certificate programs, and provided diverse rotation experiences with a large residency class. After discussions with my faculty advisor, who dually served as my mentor, I had both the confidence and expanded network to "go big or go home" with my residency pursuits. The encouragement proved to be beneficial, and I was fortunate to match to my first choice for PGY1 residency. It was during this process in which I discovered the true benefit of *mentorship*.

The *mentor-mentee relationship* is symbiotic, with the ultimate goal of both parties benefiting from a given outcome. A mentor is someone who fills in the gaps, both professionally and personally for their mentee, and assists him or her in reaching their full potential. Meanwhile, the mentee continues the legacy of lessons learned from their mentor and integrates them into their own budding mentorship style. I have realized that to raise the bar, I need my mentors to provide wisdom and guidance as I enter unchartered territory in my career. *Mentors are not there to open doors for you, but rather help you decide which door you'll need to open yourself.* Once you decide, your mentor may also be able to help you open that door more easily.

FOLLOWING THE UNDERDOG MANTRA

The second action step to help raise the bar for yourself is following a mindset that I try to teach to each of my students and residents: the *underdog mantra*. I firmly believe that success requires a deep understanding of one's confidence and humility, and the limits of each. A delicate balance exists between the two traits, and continued success often leads to a tip in the scales toward more confidence at the expense of humility. My personal check and balance between these two forces is to continually believe I am the underdog. This mindset forces you to believe that there is some other individual doing what you are trying to do, *better than you.* Accepting this assumption, however, can lead to two outcomes: self-defeat or motivation. Rather than your conscience succumbing to the former, you should be stimulated to continually think of ways to out-perform, practice better, out-teach, or out-pace others. The nature of this process automatically instills humility. Setting the bar high often leads to the creation of lofty goals. The success and confidence necessary in attaining these goals is great, but the drive to continually improve yourself—while trying to oust the elusive other "individual" performing it better—will always leave you humble, yet hungry for more.

Since starting my career as a clinical specialist, precepting has been a passion of my clinical and academic responsibilities. I was fortunate to have been inspired by many preceptors and mentors during my residency training, and I aspired to reach their status as soon as I began training students and residents. Over the past few years, I have been lucky to be recognized as a preceptor locally and nationally. Despite the recognition, however, I continually ask myself how I can be more effective. I still look up to my past preceptors and mentors as sterling examples, and find inspiration to improve my evolving preceptor style.

SEEKING OUT CHALLENGES

The last action step is germane to the act of setting the bar high for oneself. You should continually *seek out challenges*. Whether this is pursuing a residency after graduation, applying for a clinical specialist position, or pursuing a research idea that borders on landmark status, you should smile at the challenge that stands in front of you and take it head on. A major challenge I undertook during my first year as a clinical specialist was becoming the residency coordinator for our institution's PGY1 program. The role was something I aspired to, but not within the first 12 months of my career. The opportunity, however, was something that I could not pass up. Although the position presented a steep learning curve combined with a crash course in leadership, it proved to be one of the best decisions in my career. The responsibility of coordinating residents fed my passion of mentorship; two years later, I was appointed as the Assistant Program Director for our multisite PGY1 residency program. Overnight, I went from coordinating three PGY1 residents at my practice site to 11 PGY1 residents within our system—the largest program in our state.

Throughout your career, you will routinely encounter personal and professional challenges—minor or massive, cancerous, or trivial. All challenges will require action. Developing a habit of tackling them helps to build resilience and a hunger for solving problems. Although you may not defeat each challenge you encounter, the lessons gained from solving them help you scale the next metaphorical wall that is placed in front of you.

Following my diagnosis of Hodgkin's lymphoma and starting chemotherapy, I was unable to have direct patient contact for nearly eight months. My ability to effectively participate on patient care rounds and precept was challenged. Nevertheless, my residents and I developed a method to use video calling through tablets to include me in rounds without placing me at risk of infection. Failure is never final. When Thomas Edison took on the challenge of creating a long-lasting light bulb for everyday use, he was struck with a litany of failed attempts until he discovered the answer was to use a tungsten filament. When asked about his failures, he simply replied, "I have not failed 1000 times. I have successfully discovered 1000 ways to not make a light bulb."

I have discovered that hard work leads to continued success, which often generates new opportunities to expand on this success. This evolves into leadership for directing the newfound success. The profession of pharmacy is budding with opportunities to expand our role as clinicians and educators. The investment of hard work early in your career will pay off tremendously as you establish your role as a pharmacist. *Look at the bar set in front of you; how much can you raise it?*

Respectfully,

Josh

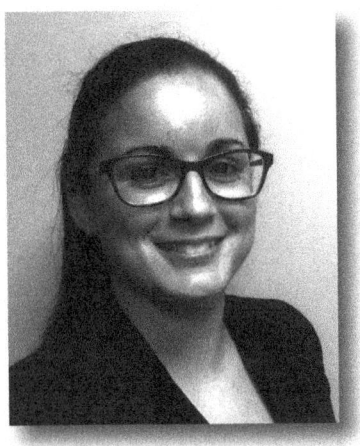

Melissa Santibañez
PharmD

Finding the Right Residencies and Making the Most of Them

Melissa is a dynamo of a young lady who is articulate and thoughtful. She had the courage to relocate twice to new places for her two residencies. She had time to write this letter while coping with Hurricane Irma and its aftermath because the college of pharmacy where she now teaches had to reschedule its classes.

Melissa is currently an Assistant Professor in Critical Care in the Department of Clinical and Administrative Sciences at Larkin University College of Pharmacy in Miami, Florida. She completed an accredited postgraduate year 1 (PGY1) pharmacy practice residency at the University of Illinois at Chicago in Chicago, Illinois, and an accredited postgraduate year 2 (PGY2) critical care residency at New York–Presbyterian Hospital in New York, New York. She received her BS in Health Sciences from the University of Miami in Coral Gables, Florida, and her PharmD from Nova Southeastern University College of Pharmacy in Fort Lauderdale, Florida.

Melissa's advice is: ***Delivering high-quality feedback was the nonclinical skill that I developed most during postgraduate training, because my preceptors gave me the tools to build constructive feedback. Remember, it's not <u>what</u> you did that matters, but <u>how</u> you did it.***

Dear Pharmacy Colleague,

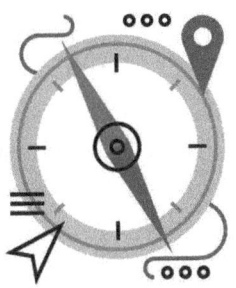

I want to start off with a story before leaving you with some words of wisdom that I've amassed since starting in hospital pharmacy nearly ten years ago but especially over the past two years during residency training. I promise there's a lesson in this, so just bear with me.

"I think what we're going to have to focus on with you is making sure that you're not bored." Those words wrapped up a

memorable interview in spring 2015 with my future PGY1 residency program director, Frank Paloucek, who was trying to figure out if I'd be an appropriate fit for the University of Illinois at Chicago (UIC) residency program. He wanted to determine if I could handle the multiple tasks and stresses that awaited me, and most importantly, if I was accepting of criticism and able to learn new skills.

That was my final PGY1 interview. Afterward, I reflected on the entire experience and every program, preceptor, and resident I'd met along the way. My immediate reaction was that UIC was the most demanding and challenging program of the bunch. It was where I could grow and develop to become an independent and capable pharmacist, and that was the atmosphere in which I wanted to train.

Since that moment, I've hearkened back to Frank's words, and I marvel at how absolutely precise his assessment was. He noticed both my potential in my need to be challenged as well as a weakness—my desire to pursue multiple projects and interests at any given time. This potential weakness could serve not only as a driving force but could also derail my career if I ever came to a point where I felt bored. At the time, I wouldn't have thought that I'd be bored especially given the fast-paced expectations of residency life that awaited me. *But, what about life after residency when you're in a fixed role and you don't get the luxury of a different clinical rotation, a new team, and a new clinical service to work with each month? What would happen when you can't essentially start fresh every month?*

By spring 2016, when I interviewed for PGY2 critical care residency positions, I used Frank's words and the general feeling I experienced during UIC as the bar against which to measure these critical care programs. I wanted the thrill of a challenge yet again while getting the best preparation I could find. When I met my future residency program director, Amy Dzierba, and explored the NewYork–Presbyterian Hospital system, I knew I'd met my match. The more I got to know her, the more I realized that she was the professional I aspired to be. Her enthusiasm and passion for critical care pharmacy reminds me of myself in many ways, and she has fueled my desire to broaden my professional horizons and get involved.

Pharmacy training is not limited to just the expansion of your clinical skills but also to the expansion of your *nonclinical* skills—the soft skills that accompany the development of a successful person.

So, my life lessons as you embark on a pharmacy career are the following:

- *Location, location, location.* Do not be afraid to take the risk of relocating away from home and to unexplored territories. This applies for both individual pharmacy school rotations and postgraduate training. Residency is not only about the pharmacy knowledge and clinical skills you will gain; it is also a new chapter in your life. The experience of living in a new place is just as important to your concept of self as the amount of information you possess. I chose to leave home for the first time for residency, and it was one of the most liberating experiences of my life. With that initial experience, I have been open to relocating based on the *caliber* of the available job opportunity. Relocation is, of course, not a limitless possibility, so careful budgeting will also determine how and when you can relocate.

- *Communicate and advocate for yourself.* Your preceptors and program directors (and co-residents!) are here to help you, but they are not omnipotent nor are they telepaths. These are extremely busy individuals with their own set of responsibilities. If you don't speak up for yourself when you believe you are being maligned or misrepresented, it may go unnoticed and the bad behavior will continue. Developing personal strength and fortitude must also accompany the development of clinical skills.

- *Seek out high-quality feedback from preceptors and faculty.* One of the most lasting skills I acquired in residency was how to give and provide feedback in a constructive way. Interestingly, too, one of the most surprising things I've noticed when precepting students and residents was how unaccustomed most young trainees are to receiving constructive criticism. A piece of feedback on how to improve is sometimes taken as an offense, when the true aim of the preceptor is to help the trainee improve and grow. Please remember, we are all human and thus imperfect. Because of that, we are *all* faced with daily opportunities to improve. One of the best parts of my PGY2 program was that we had two large academic medical centers with separate intensive care units (ICUs) as practice sites and with separate sets of critical care preceptors. My critical care preceptors were *all* committed to the residents' betterment and professional development. For every major project, they worked with me to set up practice presentations and to review my slides or handouts. The preceptors from both sites took the time to independently review my materials and provide written or verbal feedback. I sought out opportunities to work with each of them, whether for rotation or projects so I could really absorb the different skillsets they could offer me. I feel that providing quality feedback was perhaps the nonclinical skill that I developed best during residency, especially because of my PGY2 experiences.

End-of-rotation self-evaluations and quarterly evaluations were a key part of the program, and Amy made sure our evaluations answered the questions asked. She would say, "*Remember, it's not **what** you did that matters, but **how** you did it.*" Keep these questions in mind and ask yourself, "*How did I get involved with professional organizations? How did I effectively manage this complicated patient? How did my communication skills with the medical* *team change throughout this experience?"* As a trainee, an important barrier to your ability to get and provide quality feedback may be preceptors who don't openly give feedback as often as you'd like. In these cases, you must communicate your desire to be evaluated. When I encountered these situations, I found it useful to set up weekly or twice-weekly times dedicated solely to feedback and exchange, so that I could have a good working plan of what to focus on for the next week. Because of all the feedback sessions that were built into my PGY2 training, I feel extremely capable of not only precepting trainees on rotation but also of precepting and mentoring trainees on research projects and on their presentation skills. Those experiences made me a more well-rounded individual, because feedback forces you to introspect (if you're not a person already in the habit of doing so). You must objectively evaluate your performance to gauge whether the feedback you've received is valid or not. And let's not forget, many times you may find yourself in the situation of providing feedback to yourself.

- *Build your network and maintain your bridges.* I would not be in the position I'm in today without the advice of my mentors. I advise you all to find mentors and cultivate those relationships. Be aware that your mentors will evolve over time—they will be your support and lifeline throughout your training and career. Use them wisely, as these relationships are valuable and will transcend time and space. True mentorship is a two-way street; while initially you will rely more on your mentors for help, over time you will notice that those relationships will transform into collegial respect and mutual reliance.

- *Be unique.* Be an individual. Do not be a cookie cutter of everyone else or of what you think other people want you to be. Your individuality sets you apart from your competitors. (That's right! You now have competitors among your peers and colleagues: for rotations, for jobs, for fellowships, etc.) Frank admits that one of the things that drew him to my application was the opening sentence to my letter of intent in which I stated that I was a martial arts practitioner as well as a pharmacist and how the martial arts part of my life shaped my personal philosophy. It set me apart from the other applicants because it was different than the standard introduction of "I would like to sincerely express my sincerest interest in your program at _____." But then again, I've never been one to stay fully inside the lines.

- *Seek your purpose.* My professional goal in returning to South Florida after residency was to serve as a model of and advocate for progressive and autonomous pharmacist practice. South Florida has always been home to me, and I worked for many years before and during pharmacy school in various hospitals and observed hospital pharmacist practice across multiple institutions.

Regionally, as a profession, we are not as progressive and independent as we can be. I sought to bring the skills and interprofessional team dynamics (shared decision making) I had developed in both Chicago and New York to transform the pharmacy practice landscape in Florida. The best place to start is to change this culture at the level of the new generations—hence my desire to pursue academia. I can't say I would have known all this so assuredly without my multifaceted teaching experiences as a resident. Now, because my mentors opened my eyes to the possibilities that existed for me out in this big world, I find myself in a prime place to blend my clinical, teaching, and research interests to achieve that purpose.

Hopefully these words prove useful and aid your development as clinical pharmacists. Your story will not be perfect or without bumps, but please remember to make it your own and to follow your own trajectory for success. Seek your personal and professional challenges.

Melissa

Mark S. Skildum
PharmD, BCPS

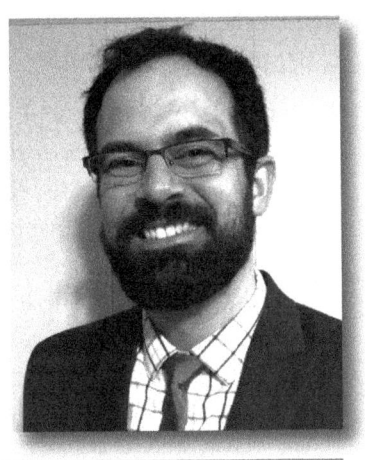

Attaining and Maximizing the Residency Experience

Mark brings his previous experiences as a teacher and coach to pharmacy leadership. He shares how he has benefited from his wife, who as an attorney, has helped him sharpen and refine his messages, and how a nursing strike provided unique residency learning experiences.

Mark is a Clinical Pharmacy Manager at United Hospital - part of Allina Health, in Saint Paul, Minnesota. He completed the ASHP Foundation's Pharmacy Leadership Academy. Mark also completed an accredited postgraduate year 1 (PGY1) pharmacy practice residency and an accredited PGY2 residency in health-system pharmacy administration at United Hospital, part of Allina Health. He received his PharmD degree from the University of Minnesota, College of Pharmacy and a BA in Biology from Saint Olaf College, Northfield, Minnesota.

Mark's advice is: *The most valuable lessons of residency are: There is something to learn from every situation and often the more challenging the situation, the more you will learn. Do not back down from difficult projects or obstacles; see them as a chance to grow.*

Dear Pharmacy Colleague,

One of my favorite sayings is "the days are long, but the years are short." Often used in the context of raising young children, I find that it applies equally well to the residency experience. In residency, your twelfth consecutive day at the hospital can feel like

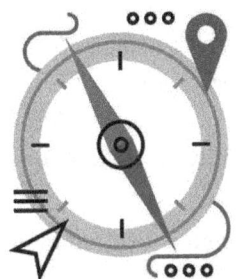

it will never end; yet, by the time you figure out what you are doing, you are already interviewing your replacement. While I can still see it clearly in the rearview mirror, I would like to share my thoughts on both attaining a residency and maximizing the residency experience. I make the disclaimer that the following tips on residency are my thoughts alone and do not necessarily reflect the views of my residency director.

KNOW YOUR WHY

During discussions with pharmacy students, they often share their desire to complete a residency and ask advice on how to attain one. They are often passionate, sharp, well-spoken, and they seek to check off all of the boxes they feel are necessary to obtain their residency. Active membership in professional organizations, *check*. Volunteering at a local free clinic, *check*. Maintaining excellent grades, *check*. A pharmacy internship at a hospital, *check*. These are the students who are doing everything they think is needed to get the residency of their dreams. The problem is that when confronted with the simple question, *why a residency?*, their usual response is a stock answer about a passion for patient care or an interest in infectious disease. Generic answers are what keep otherwise stellar candidates from standing out from the crowd. I encourage anyone applying for residency to take a hard look at your personal *why* well before application season begins. Knowing the why of your residency search will help shape both the *what* and the *how*.

I pursued pharmacy leadership because I want to positively affect the care of every hospital patient rather than limit my impact to the patients directly under my care. Crafting strategy satisfies the part of my brain that loves solving puzzles. Removing barriers and empowering others to improve and grow connects my current career to what I enjoyed most about my previous time spent as a teacher and coach.

My vision of the pharmacy leader I wanted to become was the driving force behind my choice to pursue a PGY1 followed by a PGY2 rather than a combined PGY1/2 program. Knowing that I wanted to pursue pharmacy leadership, I intended to fully focus on developing my clinical skills in my first year. My philosophy is that pharmacy leaders need to be pharmacists first. My clinical residency experiences and subsequent board certification inform my decisions when leading operational and clinical improvements. My experiences such as having a difficult conversation with a provider or patient have made me better equipped to lead and made it easier for me to hold my team accountable, while also advocating for them.

• Build Your Professional Network

Have you heard that pharmacy is a small world? As a first-year student, nothing would induce a metaphorical eye roll faster than hearing this frequently-used phrase from a preceptor or professor. However, once you hit rotations it becomes undeniable that this is the absolute truth. As a pharmacy student, building a strong network of professionals, which in turn creates future opportunities, is critical to your success. If it were not for the people in my network, my opportunities may have easily been a fraction of what I've experienced.

When building your network, the best place to start is becoming involved in one of your state pharmacy organizations. Many of these organizations offer discounted student registrations to continuing education dinners and conferences, which are a great place to meet practicing pharmacists. When you attend these meetings as a student, do not spend it huddled with your classmates—use the social time to meet someone new. Strike up conversations, ask questions about others' professional roles, positions, or area of practice; and ask them their thoughts about the areas you are passionate about. Seek insight on new or interesting areas of pharmacy that pharmacists can't seem to stop discussing. Learn their names; follow up with them next time you see them to build a relationship. *Don't ask for favors*, that's absolutely not the point. The next time you see that individual, you may then have the opportunity to meet the colleagues in his or her group. Once you establish that first relationship, each subsequent person is easier to meet because you gain the benefit of that person's network.

- ### Highlight Activities, Classes, and Rotations That Tell a Story in Your Curriculum Vitae

When preparing your curriculum vitae (CV), it is tempting to list every activity, but be concise and focus on clarity. A lengthy CV can be counterproductive and distract from your core message. Make sure your CV is not packed with filler, such as a four-line entry about a one-hour volunteering experience. A reviewer or interviewer should be able to glean a good overview of your experiences in five minutes or less.

The sum total of your experiences should lead a decision maker to understand that your involvement and experience represent your residency goals. Candidates without a roster of time spent exploring the residency area they seek may appear to be undereducated, which can cause doubt or questioning over the candidate's understanding or dedication to this area of practice. Decision makers want candidates with a full knowledge of the field they are pursuing, while demonstrating commitment and the ability to "stay the course" during the challenges of residency.

The story I wanted to tell during my residency application process was that of a pharmacy student with a deep interest in both hospital pharmacy leadership and clinical pharmacy. I emphasized my rotations and electives that fit this narrative and minimized or removed entirely activities that were not relevant. I highlighted accomplishments and interests such as the student board liaison to our state chapter of ASHP and my leadership classes, and I deleted items such as a single-year membership in managed care and consulting pharmacy national organizations.

- ### Keep Track of Your Stories and Experiences

Many employers use behavior-based questions for both residency and staff position interviews. These are questions that often start with "tell me about a time..." or "describe a situation...." One of the best ways to prepare for this is to keep track of memorable experiences that happen at school, on rotation, or at work. This could be anything from a spiral notebook to an indexed collection in a cloud-based note-taking program (Evernote is my personal favorite). The key is recording a quick summary of the situation and what kind of question it fits best. For example, if you had a very busy night at your internship, the entry could read: *Busy night on the intern shift, many priorities to juggle, was able to triage phone calls effectively and get the TPA run down to the ED quickly. Team worked really well together.* The night before an interview, review your stories and reflect back on the situation. This will ensure you are prepared with great examples of teamwork, conflict, or juggling priorities.

- ### Have Someone from Outside of Pharmacy Read All Application Materials and Critique Your Presentations

Many pharmacy students have a background in the sciences and possess an ability to write clearly and succinctly. The drawback of this more technical writing style is that it can lead to a lack of emotion and voice when you are writing a letter of intent or preparing for an interview.

My wife is an attorney and writes for a living. Having her eyes on my work refines my focus, adds value, and increases the overall quality of my message. Nonetheless, to benefit from this process, the critique must be honest and your reviewer must be invested in your success. If you have such a person, congratulations—the battle is half won. If you don't have someone outside of pharmacy you are comfortable approaching, find an alternative; perhaps another pharmacy student eager to enjoy a reciprocal benefit. My closest pharmacy school classmate and I spent many hours reviewing and rehearsing applications and questions; I benefited greatly from this pharmacy background sounding board.

DURING RESIDENCY: RISE TO THE OCCASION

As my PGY1 residency year was ending, the nurses' union representing the nurses at the three large hospitals in my health system called a seven-day strike. Pharmacy leaders from across our health system outlined a number of steps that would be taken to support our new temporary nurses and ensure the safety and quality of care provided to our patients. In addition, the management team at my hospital outlined their goals for how to best support our temporary nursing work force. My director tasked my three co-residents and me with three priorities: the management of all medication protocols; the creation of resource documents for the nurses; and extending decentralized pharmacy services in our emergency department and intensive care units. Leading up to the week of the strike, my co-residents and I developed a plan that met all of our management team's objectives. As intensity and pressure mounted, we jokingly referred to it as our final exam week; as it grew closer, we felt a nervous excitement for what was to come. I began the week as the overnight resource pharmacist, providing additional "at the elbow" support to our new teammates in the emergency department and intensive care units. Another co-resident and I volunteered to staff these overnight shifts to ensure coverage during the transition.

After two months passed without a contract between the nurses' union and the hospital, the nurses began an open-ended strike that lasted 37 days. This brought new challenges to procedures and protocols. Again, we did what was needed to ensure patient safety, taking the lessons learned from the seven-day strike and applying them to a strike without a defined end. The stability of our traveling nurse workforce allowed our department to gradually return to normal operations. As the nurses grew comfortable and learned hospital procedures, we were able to transition more tasks back to them. This transition plan was a unique opportunity; we had to make difficult decisions on how and when to shift responsibility, as well as how to educate the nurses and ensure their ability to complete tasks as we shifted responsibilities from pharmacy back to nursing. In retrospect, although it was a monumental and consuming task, this second strike was one of the most valuable experiences of my second year of residency because I capitalized on the opportunities presented to me.

This is one of the most valuable lessons of residency: There is something to learn from every situation and often the more challenging the situation, the more you will learn. Do not back down from difficult projects or obstacles; see them as a chance to grow.

What I gained from residency was much more than expanded medication knowledge or management skills. Residency is about developing the thought process and personal organizational skills to tackle any problem presented. There are inevitably setbacks and challenges in any residency year, but those are the experiences that help you evolve into a better clinician and leader.

Best,

Mark

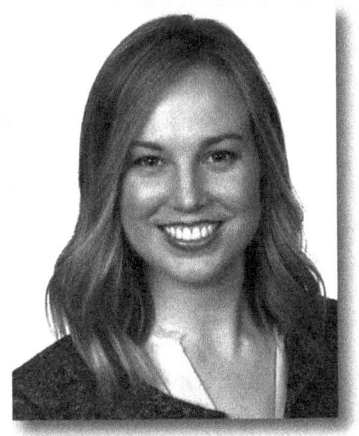

Katherine M. Smith
PharmD, BCACP

Dream Big and Seek Mentors to Guide You Along the Way

Katie came from a family of pharmacists and really did not want to continue the trend. However, after working as a pharmacy technician in a compounding pharmacy, she was convinced that she should continue her family's legacy in the pharmacy profession. Along her journey she met several mentors who influenced her career in many ways until she found her "dream" career position.

Katie is currently a Clinical Assistant Professor at the University of Houston College of Pharmacy. She received her PharmD degree from Creighton University School of Pharmacy and Health Professions in Omaha, Nebraska. She then completed her postgraduate year 1 (PGY1) pharmacy practice residency and PGY2 ambulatory care pharmacy residency at the Michael E. DeBakey Veterans Affairs (VA) Medical Center in Houston, Texas. She maintains an ambulatory care clinical practice at a federally qualified health center, Vecino Health Centers–Denver Harbor Family Clinic, where she manages chronic disease states through prescriptive authority under a collaborative practice agreement and precepts fourth year advanced pharmacy practice experience (APPE) students.

Katie's advice is: ***Dream big, seek out mentors that guide you and cheer for your success, and then follow through by precepting and mentoring future pharmacy students.***

Dear Pharmacy Colleague,

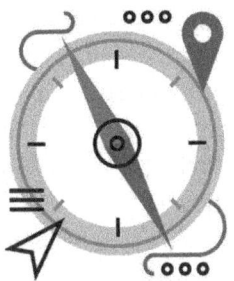

Upon and even prior to graduation from pharmacy school, one constant question running through your mind may have been, "*In which direction do I want to steer my career?*" The field of pharmacy has countless facets and limitless opportunities for a successful career, which is what originally drew me to the profession, but those limitless opportunities can also be overwhelming. However, I learned that each experience within the pharmacy world will shape the direction of your career, and countless mentors along the way will help guide and believe in your aspirations.

FOLLOWING THE FAMILY CAREER PATHS INTO PHARMACY

Pharmacy was engrained in me at an early age. My mother is a pharmacist. She has held multiple roles throughout her career, including working with oncology and HIV patients, serving as an infusion pharmacist, and currently working as an Associate Director of Pharmacy Operations for a pharmaceutical company and specialty pharmacy. My great uncle, uncle, and now a cousin own the only pharmacy in the small town of Windsor, Missouri.

When asked at a young age about my career aspirations, I would give generic answers such as a teacher or a soccer player. However, I would also say that I absolutely did not want to become a pharmacist like the rest of my family. This thought changed when I was in high school and started working as a pharmacy technician for Stark Pharmacy, a compounding pharmacy, in Overland Park, Kansas. I admired the relationships the pharmacists established with their patients. We compounded hormones into many dosage forms including capsules, troches, and creams. The pharmacists met with patients to review hormone levels and symptoms. They would often contact the physician and recommend a change in hormone dosage that we were compounding for the patient. From that point on, I had a desire to pursue a career as an ambulatory care pharmacist. I wanted to create the same relationships with patients and have a significant impact on patient care. The pharmacy's owner saw my spark of interest for this profession and invested in me. He allowed me to take on many roles as a technician so I could garner the most experience and observe all of the pharmacist's responsibilities in this setting. He, along with my family of pharmacists, was my first mentor.

SEEKING OUT MENTORS

During pharmacy school, I sought out ambulatory care faculty mentors and activities that would further expose me to ambulatory care pharmacy in addition to other areas of pharmacy. Because my mother had the opportunity to pursue different tracks within the profession during her career, I wanted to also explore multiple roles available to a pharmacist. Volunteering in numerous interprofessional health fairs and participating in two medical mission trips to the Dominican Republic solidified my desire to become an ambulatory care pharmacist. Transitioning into residency, I credit wonderful preceptors who gave their time and provided me with important tips to overcoming the challenges and obstacles I was facing on the path to achieving my goals. For example, they gave me advice about how to be more efficient in completing daily clinical tasks. They went to great lengths to arrange a meeting with the Chief of Cardiology so I could pitch my research idea. My preceptors reminded me to focus not only on gaining the most knowledge I could to become an excellent ambulatory care pharmacist, but to develop the skills necessary to design a patient-centered clinical practice. One of my preceptors even had a physician new to the practice "shadow" me so that I could demonstrate the value of a pharmacist in a primary care clinic—a lesson I continue to utilize today.

AN IMPACTFUL MENTOR

One key mentor in my career has been my PGY1 Residency Program Director (RPD), Dr. Richard M. Cadle. I admired his passion and persistence for advocating at the state and national level for the pharmacy profession in expanding clinical pharmacy services. His ultimate passion was investing in the training and future careers of pharmacy students and residents and inspired them to set high goals and pursue their dream careers. He spent time daily getting to know our passions and desires, guide us through challenges, provide honest feedback, and be our cheerleader. Even though he was not my RPD for my PGY2 residency in ambulatory care, his mentorship did not stop. He credited himself as my "second RPD" because he was still invested in my success.

After learning about an opening for my dream job during my PGY2 residency, I contemplated applying but decided to pursue it later on in my career. When Dr. Cadle heard about this position and that I did not intend to apply, he came directly to the resident office and gave me a clever ultimatum. I had to apply for this position that evening or he would not allow me to come to work the next day. Now, this seemed like a pretty good deal to an often overloaded resident. But that is not how he saw it; instead, he gave me the confidence to apply and reiterated his faith in me that I would succeed in this position. He told me this position sounded exactly like the ideal position I had been describing to him throughout my two years of residency. It encompassed my desire for precepting and teaching (a passion I had learned about myself under his supervision) in an interprofessional ambulatory care setting with the patient population with which I wanted to make a difference. I believe this situation perfectly summarizes his traits as an exemplary mentor over two years—guiding me with passion while being my cheerleader, yet providing honest feedback when needed regarding my fit into this position versus others. From that point forward, I have sought to emulate these traits as I mentor future pharmacists.

ADVOCATING FOR OUR PROFESSION AND IMPARTING ADVICE

Dr. Cadle's untimely passing happened six months after I started working at my new dream position. His passing left a void. However, one thing that I and many of his trainees could take solace in is our ability to impart his advice to future students and trainees. Another of his lessons that I carried with me to my current position is advocating for the profession and expanding the role of pharmacists. In his career, he had expanded the clinical pharmacy department at the Houston VA from only a pair of pharmacists to over 30 pharmacists. As a resident, I worked with him to create a business plan for a pharmacist in the women's clinic. This experience gave me the skills to start a new clinical pharmacy service at my ambulatory care practice site, a family medicine clinic where there had not been a pharmacist in over two years. Many other former residents have paved the way in expanding the role for pharmacists, which includes creating a new antimicrobial stewardship service, forming a transitions of care team, and establishing other ambulatory care services.

His impact was far-reaching, and now I have the opportunity to continue that impact through my own mentorship. I remember the trust and desire for guidance that I placed in my mentors, so I consider this perspective when I am mentoring pharmacy students. In the skills labs that I facilitate or student organizations I am involved with, I have tried to demonstrate how I want to assist in student success. Many students have scheduled meetings with me so that we can discuss their desires and develop a plan to achieve them. I have found joy in noticing the strengths of a student who did not realize them herself, providing honest feedback during her rotation so that she utilized those strengths to exceed expectations, and cheering her on while she applied to multiple pharmacist positions. Another student happily informed me that she has decided to pursue ambulatory care after shadowing me in clinic, asking for more guidance in this pharmacy track. My hope is that the mentoring skills I have developed from my mentors will also be passed along through the students I teach. Recounting the steps in my journey reminds me that each experience has shaped and directed my career. I went from never wanting to be a pharmacist at an early age to a new practitioner loving the emerging career I have now. I am working where I am today because of Dr. Cadle and countless other mentors along the way. I will continue their legacy by mentoring pharmacy students and residents and advocating for the profession.

As you begin your career, remember:

- **Dream big. It is not too early to pursue your dream career.** The experiences that you have along the way are vital to shaping and directing your future career.

- **Seek out mentors who guide your passion and cheer for your success.** Identify a pharmacist who is invested in your future and will listen to your goals. Ask for honest advice as you navigate your career path. There should be no limit on the number of mentors you may have during your career or at a given time. When transitioning jobs, notice the pharmacists who go out of their way to ensure you are succeeding in your new role; they may become your new mentors.

- **Become a preceptor and mentor to pharmacy students**. As your career matures, you become transformed solely from being the *mentee* to becoming a *mentor* for others. Yet, during the process you still retain your special relationship with your own mentors. Provide the same, excellent mentorship you received in your young career. Providing such guidance to others will include advocacy for the profession, so we, as pharmacists, can provide the best patient-centered care possible.

Best wishes in your future career!

Sincerely,

Katie

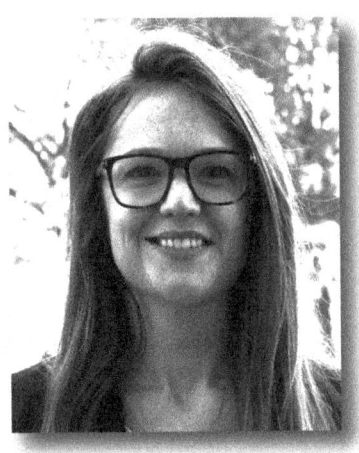

Jessica Snead
PharmD, BCGP

Pursue Your Passion

Jessica was determined to complete a postgraduate year 1 (PGY1) residency. With grit and doggedness, her determination paid off in spades for Montefiore Medical Center as she became one of their PGY1 residents in 2015. They were fortunate to mentor an enthusiastic, driven, and engaging individual who went on to complete a PGY2 residency in internal medicine.

Jessica is currently Clinical Pharmacy Manager, Internal Medicine, New York–Presbyterian Hospital, Weill Cornell Medical Center, New York, New York. Jessica completed her accredited PGY2 internal medicine pharmacy residency at Kingsbrook Jewish Medical Center, Brooklyn, New York and her accredited PGY1 pharmacy residency at Montefiore Medical Center, The Bronx, New York. Jessica received her PharmD degree at Virginia Commonwealth University, Richmond and her BS in Biological Sciences, North Carolina State University, Raleigh.

Jessica's advice is: **Finding your passion is the most important aspect of your career—having fulfillment in your profession is why we all pursue pharmacy.**

Dear Pharmacy Colleague,

Completing my residency training has by far been the most exciting two years of my

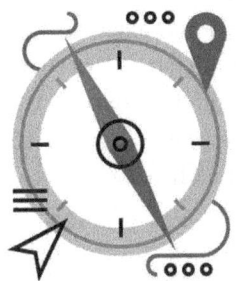

life. The exponential degree of learning and the challenges that you face are unlike any you will ever experience again. During the days and nights I spent in training, I made lifelong friends, connected with professional colleagues, and developed camaraderie with co-residents that can never be replaced. The mentorship and training I received throughout residency made me the clinical pharmacist I am today and helped me carve the path to my professional career.

During pharmacy school, I began to discover the aspects of the profession that I was most passionate about. As I became familiar with faculty who had completed residency training, I was amazed by the way they practiced medicine and their clinical knowledge of pathological disease states. My favorite professor completed his residency training in geriatrics and led a volunteer clinic that focused on interdisciplinary team rounding with an underserved geriatric population. This was my first exposure to seeing how medicine, social work, nursing, and pharmacy can efficiently collaborate to make comprehensive healthcare plans for special populations. The impact and the quality of care patients received through this collaboration motivated me to start considering residency. Additionally, watching my older pharmacy school acquaintances complete residencies and seeing them grow clinically was inspiring. Looking back, I was fortunate during pharmacy school to be surrounded by mentors and role models who encouraged me to further hone my skills through residency.

IMPORTANT LESSONS AND PIVOTAL MOMENTS

The most practical and important lessons I learned in pharmacy were gained during my fourth year in advanced pharmacy practice experiences (APPEs). I took every opportunity to complete rotations with broad experiences, interesting patient populations, and preceptors who were experts in their specialty area. My internal medicine APPE was in a large academic medical center in southwestern Virginia. I spent all waking hours in the hospital following general medicine patients. This is where I was first taught how to apply the pharmaceutical knowledge we learn in school to a practical situation and to think critically about medical therapy. The patient population in this area had low health literacy, and I saw how pharmacists made an impact on a patient's therapy through medication reconciliation, participating in daily rounds, and discharge counseling. I even had the opportunity to see a paracentesis. I'll never forget this because I fainted during the procedure, and my preceptor caught me in mid-air.

Another pivotal APPE was an Indian Health Service (IHS) rotation in Northeastern Arizona. Out of the numerous applicants, I was lucky enough to draw Chinle, Arizona in the Navajo Nation! I lived in a double-wide trailer on the compound with rotating obstetrics/gynecology (OB/GYN) medical residents. This was the only healthcare facility within hundreds of miles. They cared for a diverse range of patients. I saw my first of many *Mycobacterium tuberculosis* and necrotizing fasciitis cases on the reservation. The IHS pharmacy department was inclusive with pharmacy students and always utilized them on their projects. For example, I completed a surveillance study on *Clostridium difficile* and collaborated on an article for the IHS journal. Most importantly, I learned about the health disparity that exists and the opportunity for a pharmacist to help patients who live in a rural area with limited healthcare access. Both of these APPE experiences influenced my decision to seek out residencies that provided healthcare to an underserved population. I later matched to programs in The Bronx and Brooklyn, New York.

Through these APPE experiences, I knew my ultimate goal would be to match with a residency program. To achieve this goal, getting involved with professional organizations both locally and nationally was essential for networking. Attending the Personnel Placement Service (PPS) during the ASHP Midyear Clinical Meeting was also important in the years leading up to and during residency. The interviews and networking during those events led me to residency interviews, job interviews, and actual job offers. New York City has an excellent local chapter for hospital pharmacists who promote our profession through volunteer work, collaborating on continuing education courses with pharmaceutical companies, and even working on grass-roots lobbying for pharmacy initiatives. This is where my co-residents and I did most of our networking, and I continue to be an active member as a clinical pharmacist. I can't emphasize enough how pharmacy is such a small world and how making connections with your colleagues at any opportunity is essential.

As a southern girl from Virginia, I learned many lessons during my residency in The Bronx—the first was not to make eye contact on the subway or any public space in New York City. In the hospital pharmacy, I learned many lessons on leadership, organizational prioritization, and clinical knowledge that never would have been possible without exposure to residency training. During my first year of residency, I completed my staffing requirement by acting as both the Operations Manager and narcotic pharmacist every other weekend and on holidays. My first weekend working alone the local power company accidently cut a wire, which jeopardized electricity to the entire hospital. I quickly learned where the flashlights were kept and how important generators are for large health systems. In January, there was a 27-inch blizzard that shut down the entire city. Public transportation was halted, and all streets and highways were closed for non-emergent travel. The connections I made while validating medication orders in near-complete darkness and having five pharmacists stay in my fifth floor walk-up apartment overnight led to making lifelong friends.

One of my most memorable clinical rotations during my first year of residency was with the renal transplant pharmacist. We counseled patients on their new immunosuppressant regimen, and she taught me the importance of attention to detail which I witnessed first-hand in monitoring a transplant patient's recovery and progress. We tightly monitored and adjusted medications for their blood pressure, glycemic control, and tacrolimus levels. I completed my first residency presentations with her, began my research projects, and even had the opportunity to watch a 6-hour renal transplant surgery. The Medical Intensive Care Unit rotation was another milestone rotation. My preceptor had a longstanding relationship with the attending physicians, which made it easy for pharmacy residents to become part of the medical teaching rounds. This was my first experience in a diverse urban hospital that handled high acuity patient presentations, from acute liver failure to coccidioidal meningitis. I'll never forget when a status epilepticus patient who was on high doses of propofol, midazolam, and other sedatives came back to the hospital to bring the team doughnuts. Seeing a patient intubated then walking and talking the next week is one of my most precious memories and reminds me of the importance of maximizing every patient's medication therapy to improve outcomes.

My decision to continue into a second year of residency was simple: I wanted to be the clinical pharmacist with the clinical acumen I saw in my mentors. Their ability to improve patient outcomes and hospital pharmacy practices was something I had come to idolize. My second year was spent in a community hospital in Brooklyn completing an internal medicine residency. The gratitude of the underserved patient population for a pharmacist was a daily motivation. Most of the patients were immigrants who had never received formal healthcare. The management of chronic, untreated conditions and acute infections was both challenging and rewarding. I formed personal relationships with many patients through a quality project on improving medication adherence in heart failure. When patients actively participated in their healthcare, it directly led to better outcomes. Counseling and communicating with patients effectively about their medications at any point is essential for their therapy. That important point— that a pharmacist in any setting can have a huge impact on this aspect of healthcare— was made again and again during the rotation.

Serving as a mentor is another concept that has been ingrained in me. Whether it was as a student, resident, or clinical pharmacist, having a mentor or role model has been vital to my personal and professional development. It is essential for our profession to continually encourage and develop future pharmacists. I encourage you to be the kind of mentor who inspires pharmacy students to pursue their passion (and catch them if they fall). Even in pharmacy school, you can serve as a mentor to the younger classes. As I previously mentioned, my upperclassmen inspired me to pursue residency. I completed a teaching certificate at a local pharmacy school, precepted pharmacy students in the hospital, and helped coordinate a pharmacy laboratory course during both years of my residencies. I can't emphasize enough how special it has been to see pharmacy students reach their goals. I had several students in my second year of residency who went on to match in their top-ranked programs. This has been the most rewarding part of my career so far, and I am excited to see where their careers will take them.

My first position after residency is an Internal Medicine Clinical Pharmacy Manager at a large academic medical center in New York City. The dedication to both my PGY1 and 2 clinical training directly prepared me for this current role. I follow between 15–20 general medicine patients daily and round with the multidisciplinary medical team. There is a large emphasis on transitions of care. I ensure each patient has a thorough medication reconciliation completed on admission and discharge counseling. Improving and developing discharge counseling on chronic obstructive pulmonary disease (COPD), diabetes, heart failure, and anticoagulation medication therapy is one of my passions. A large focus now is to streamline the process by utilizing technology to complete all medication reconciliations through tele-health.

ABOVE ALL, PASSION IS KEY

Ultimately, I encourage pharmacy students to pursue their passion. How can you improve medication therapy and outcomes for patients? What will challenge you in a way that makes you improve on your skillset and knowledge continually? Finding that passion is by far the most important aspect of your career—having fulfillment in your profession is why we all pursue pharmacy. It is my hope that residency programs throughout the country continue to expand, and that there are enough programs for the number of pharmacy students graduating each year. *Pursuing residency was the best decision I ever made. I challenge and encourage every pharmacy student to complete one too.*

Kind regards,

Jess

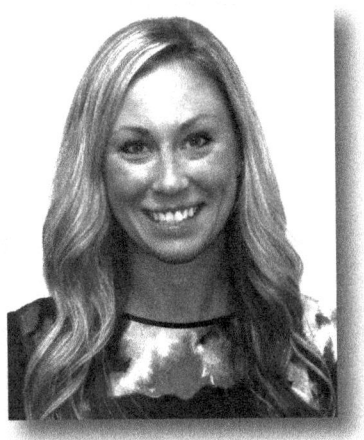

Laura K. Triantafylidis
PharmD

Go into a Pharmacy Setting and Leave It Better Than When You Started

Laura is committed to ensuring that her patients receive the best possible care. She routinely goes the extra step to ensure that no details are overlooked. Whether it is a follow-up phone call, a meeting with a caregiver, or walking a patient to his next appointment, Laura is always available to help.

Laura is currently a Clinical Pharmacy Specialist for Women's Health and Community Based Outpatient Clinics at VA Boston Healthcare System in Massachusetts. Laura completed an accredited postgraduate year 1 (PGY1) pharmacy residency at Lahey Hospital and Medical Center, Burlington, Massachusetts, and an accredited PGY2 geriatrics pharmacy specialty residency at the VA Boston Healthcare System. She received her PharmD, BS in Pharmacy Studies, and BS in Allied Health from the University of Connecticut, Storrs.

Laura's advice is: *Take chances and allow yourself to experience new and exciting areas of pharmacy, don't be afraid to change your mind or pursue the path you least expected, and take advantage of all the opportunities that come your way.*

Dear Pharmacy Colleague,

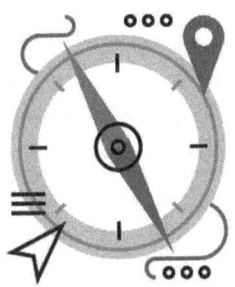

It feels like just yesterday that I was a first-year pharmacy student. If you had asked me six years ago where I imagined my pharmacy career would go, I would have never imagined I would take the path I traveled. Initially, I anticipated a career in the retail setting. I worked in retail prior to and during pharmacy school, and I loved the patient–provider interaction. My early experiences led me to believe the drugstore setting represented the typical pharmacist career. To be honest, at the start of pharmacy school, I had never even heard of a pharmacy residency and knew little about how pharmacists functioned in the hospital or clinical setting.

My first hospital experience was during my second year as a pharmacy student when I was placed at a tertiary teaching hospital with more than 800 beds. As you can imagine, coming from a small retail pharmacy in a grocery store, this was a huge change. During this experience, I learned as much as I could about what it meant to be a clinical pharmacy specialist. I shadowed various specialty areas including critical care, pain management, cardiology, and infectious disease. I loved it all. It was an eye-opening experience, and I quickly discovered the endless opportunities that existed for pharmacists.

NEW EXPERIENCES TRANSLATE TO CHANGING INTERESTS

My interest in hospital pharmacy grew throughout the remainder of pharmacy school. During my last year, my first advanced pharmacy practice experience (APPE) was a three-month longitudinal rotation at a large teaching hospital where I rotated through cardiology, critical care, and internal medicine learning experiences. In some ways, it was like a mini-residency. During these rotations, I became very comfortable in the hospital setting, and I realized pursuing a residency would help me obtain the job that best suited me.

My first instinct to help improve my chances at gaining a residency position was to become more involved in the profession and more well-rounded by demonstrating varied interests and abilities. To me, that meant getting my hands on a project that would be worthy of presentation at the student poster session at the 2014 ASHP Midyear Clinical Meeting. While in search of a project and brainstorming ideas, one of my mentors gave me a great piece of advice that stuck with me: "*Always go into a pharmacy setting and try to leave it better than when you started.*" I have carried this advice with me whether it involves optimizing the use of a medication, dispensing or handling medications, or providing patient care. There is always room for improvement and innovation.

Fast-forward a few months, and it was time to prepare for the residency match and to rank residency programs. This was going to be one of the most important decisions I ever had to make, yet I was still unsure about so many things. I had questions such as: *Will my residency determine where I end up in my career? Do I have to pick an area of specialty now? What if I have to move or relocate?* There were so many questions, and so few answers. I had to resort back to what I *did* know. I knew I wanted to learn as much as possible to excel in the clinical setting and provide direct patient care, and I had a strong passion for teaching and learning. I sought advice from my well-respected mentors. I asked them about their career paths and training experiences. A PGY2 pharmacy resident who co-precepted me during an APPE rotation was very helpful. I felt my career goals were aligned with hers and truly valued her encouragement to pursue residency. Additionally, one of my mentors who had completed a PGY1 and PGY2 emphasized the importance of a residency. He advised me to pursue a residency if I wanted a career in hospital pharmacy because it would provide experiences beyond those available in pharmacy school and prepare me to function independently as a clinical pharmacist. Fortunately, I ended up at a program that aligned with my interests and goals—a tertiary teaching, community hospital that supported inpatient and outpatient clinical experiences.

After graduating pharmacy school, things started to move at full speed. I acquired my pharmacy license and started my first "real" job—a PGY1 pharmacy residency. I quickly learned that residency is a journey. I looked at my residency as an investment in my future. Going into residency, you must keep in mind you are there to learn and grow. You are not going to know everything, but you will be pushed to learn quickly!

ENDLESS OPPORTUNITIES AWAIT IN RESIDENCY

One of the best things in residency is the seemingly endless opportunities it provides. Do you think you have an interest in infectious disease, but you aren't sure? OK—go spend a month with the infectious disease clinical pharmacist. Have you decided infectious disease isn't right for you, but you think you might prefer managing hypertension/diabetes in the ambulatory setting? Spend the next month with the ambulatory care clinical pharmacist. The beauty of residency is that it offers the time to experience and learn as many different things as possible. Hopefully, in the end, it will give you the knowledge and tools to decide with confidence what area of pharmacy suits you best.

I went into residency thinking I wanted to pursue a specialty in critical care. Three months into my program, I had a complete change of heart. After completing a medical intensive care unit (ICU) rotation, I moved on to an internal medicine rotation. There was a definite change of pace from rounding in the ICU with very sick, intubated patients to rounding on the floors spending face-to-face time with patients. I deliberately took on the role of providing patients and family members discharge medication education. I spent time with newly diagnosed diabetics teaching them how to inject insulin, heart failure exacerbation patients who had difficulty with medication adherence, and elderly patients who had difficulty managing their complex medication regimens. I enjoyed spending time with patients and family members and helping them to better understand their medications for improved disease state management. I realized how much I missed the day-to-day patient interaction and decided I preferred a setting that allowed me to develop strong patient relationships. Having known I wanted to further my training with a PGY2 pharmacy residency, I decided to pursue a geriatrics pharmacy residency. I could continue to gain experiences in inpatient and outpatient settings while working directly with a unique patient population with complex comorbidities and multiple medications that would benefit greatly from pharmacist involvement.

Aside from the broad range of experiences that residency afforded, it also allowed me to become involved with worthy clinical research and quality improvement projects. Residency supports dedicated time to projects that will improve clinical practice and allow for process improvement. It is an excellent opportunity to learn from those with expertise in these areas, gain practical experience, and share your work with others in the field through clinical meetings and professional conferences.

Although my journey through residency ended just three short months ago, my journey as a clinical pharmacy specialist has merely just begun. I feel fortunate to be in the role that I am in today, and I use my training and work experiences daily to provide optimal patient care.

I want to end with some pieces of advice for future pharmacists: (1) take chances and allow yourself to experience new and exciting areas of pharmacy, (2) don't be afraid to change your mind or pursue the path you least expected, and (3) take advantage of all the opportunities that come your way because you never know if they will come along again.

Sincerely,

Laura

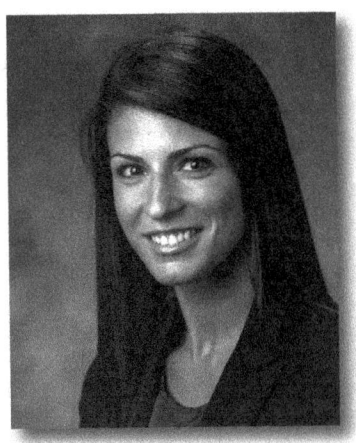

Allison M. Vecchiet
PharmD, MS

Maximizing Life's Transitions

Allison is a risk taker who hustles to make the most out of every experience and is not afraid to choose the road less traveled. You will learn from her letter how she handled important transitions to guide her professional career and continue to perfect herself.

Allison is currently a Pharmacy Consulting Director with Huron Consulting Group, Chicago, Illinois. She completed an accredited postgraduate year 1 (PGY1) pharmacy practice residency and accredited PGY2 health-system pharmacy administration residency at Nationwide Children's Hospital, Columbus, Ohio. Allison received a BS in Biochemistry from DeSales University, Center Valley, Pennsylvania and her PharmD and MS in Health-System Pharmacy Administration from The Ohio State University, College of Pharmacy, Columbus.

Allison's advice is: ***Throughout your career, you will constantly face tough decisions and critical transition points. Set yourself up for success by seeking out mentors, following your trajectory, embracing your failures, and stepping outside of your comfort zone.***

Dear Pharmacy Colleague,

Successful pharmacy leaders have career paths filled with events where a thoughtful deci-

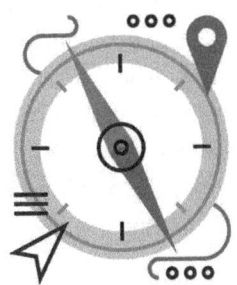

sion was made in response to a high-stakes transition. Some of those transitions are self-driven, while others are decided upon from different forces. Some transitions are simply necessary changes while others are critical reflection points. I hope that this collection of personal transitions empowers you to confidently respond to the transitions that will shape your career path as a pharmacy leader.

FOLLOW YOUR TRAJECTORY

Pop-culture-themed chemistry demonstrations, gold nanoparticles, and a few inspiring leaders were the (not-so-obvious) factors that took me from being a wide-eyed biochemistry undergraduate to a PharmD/PhD graduate student 500 miles away from home! Undergrad was a time to hustle in and out of the classroom, but simultaneously a time to **not** take life too seriously. For me, it translated in a debut science demonstration program that allowed me to teach high school students about chemistry using pop culture references. It also meant that my senior research project would be the study of electrochemistry of gold nanoparticles because I really liked chemistry and gold, equally! More importantly, the mentors who surrounded me during this time were diverse and accomplished leaders in pharmacy, medicine, and the sciences. I approached senior year with big ambitions and equal uncertainties. So, I cast my net wide and decided to pursue a PharmD/PhD Translational Science program at The Ohio State University (OSU), which captured my interests to be both a clinician and a scientist. At the time, I made the choice because I couldn't be decisive. In retrospect, this transition was one of the greatest reflection points in my career because it taught me the value of following my trajectory.

During pharmacy school, I was fortunate enough to be selected for an administrative internship at the College of Pharmacy to support, manage, and grow the Latiolais Leadership Program for OSU's combined Master of Science (MS)/residency in health-system pharmacy administration. At the time, I knew very little about pharmacy administration, and I was the first intern for the program. Without a precedent or an example to follow, it was an intimidating and refreshingly humbling experience to be surrounded by a group of accomplished alumni who had made many lasting impacts on our profession. I was in awe of their drive and passion for leadership, our profession, and fortunately for me, developing others. My boss and the other Executive Steering Committee members encouraged me to use my unique strengths and to raise my hand even when I didn't think I had anything to contribute. They gave me the opportunity to create new programming, branding, and communication strategies. This experience made me realize that I thrived in settings that required me to be self-driven, innovative, and as my boss would say, "deliver the message to Garcia." The tremendous personal and professional satisfaction from this internship experience, as well as my leadership roles with student government and pharmacy organizations, led me to leave the doctorate (PhD) portion of my program. This was a difficult decision because no one likes to "quit," but my strengths, network of mentors and coaches, and my gradually emerging passions for strategy and organizational management did not align with completing a PhD. Following my momentum, I chose to complete my PharmD and pursue a combined MS/residency in health-system pharmacy administration.

Following my trajectory has since led me to hold several leadership positions in and out of pharmacy; it guided my decision to pursue a pharmacy residency; and it drove me to follow a nontraditional and rewarding career path. No matter where you are in your career, I challenge you to find your trajectory and respond to your next major transition with a decision that follows this momentum.

Reflect on the environments and skillsets where you succeeded better than your peers and pick the path that will put you in that environment. Going through this process can help you be more decisive when presented with a difficult transition and will give you the confidence to succeed during an uncertain time.

LISTEN. LEARN. REFLECT. REPEAT.

Pharmacists will all face humbling and impressionable events in their careers. Failed exams, rigorous rotations, and residency match heartbreak are just a few of the events that you can relate to or expect to face. Humbling experiences are a unique opportunity to listen to tough feedback, learn what you did wrong, and reflect on how you will respond differently next time. Emotions make this difficult at first, but over time you will learn to respect the feedback and embrace it as an opportunity to critically change. This sounds obvious, but it is not easy to implement! When I started my combined MS/residency, I was immediately met with rigorous clinical rotations, evening classes, weekend staffing, and longitudinal project commitments. Preceptors, teachers, and mentors held me to a high standard regardless of my competing priorities. Stress was mounting, but these feelings were not unfamiliar. Over four years in pharmacy school, I managed coursework, research, and an internship; I also spent two years as Secretary and President of OSU's graduate student body. Competing priorities forced me to communicate frequently with colleagues whom I relied on to move along action items. Diverse project work forced me to identify bottlenecks early, especially for situations where I was at risk for being the bottleneck.

Most importantly, my experiences in pharmacy school toughened me to tolerate and perform in high-stress environments without compromising quality. Residency was hard, but I never under-delivered and always tried to exceed expectations because of the emotional growth I developed from four years of listening, learning, and reflecting. The best way to apply this is to think of a time when you made the same mistake twice. Consider how circumstances may have changed the second time around if you had been intentional in reflecting after the first mistake. Decide now how you will implement this step-wise process the next time you make a mistake.

BREAK BOUNDARIES

Journals, conferences, and professional organizations are platforms for pharmacists to advance the profession in solidarity. Be an active contributor in these forums and always invest in your professional growth. The best way to contribute in these forums is to bring interdisciplinary solutions that come from your experience working outside of the pharmacy realm. Technology and information consumption is shifting the practice of pharmacy every day. The role of the pharmacist is expanding in response to these changes, and attention is increasingly directed toward pharmacy leaders who bring more than just a PharmD to the table.

During my time with OSU's graduate student government, I worked with a design major who inspired me by his ability to apply beautiful elements of design to rebrand an organization, communicate information digitally, and display complex data. I admired this skill for its application in pharmacy. Immediately, I began applying many aspects of thoughtful design to pharmacy deliverables in work and school and eventually in residency and now in my career as a consultant. This has allowed me to communicate very complicated content in a familiar and approachable way. This also allows me to convey pharmacy solutions to hospital leaders with very different backgrounds in a digestible format that is clinically and financially rigorous.

Look in unexpected places for inspiration that can enhance the pharmacy profession and focus this outward view toward areas where you have strengths. You will increase your marketability as a pharmacy leader if you can bring new ideas or new approaches to solve persistent pharmacy problems.

I hope some of my experiences or suggestions encourage you to reflect on your current trajectory. If not, reread these letters when you transition into the next phase of your life. I have found this to be incredibly useful! After each transition, I spend time getting acclimated to my new role and the organization's culture. Without fail, an event, challenge, or interaction will trigger my memory and I'll recall a piece of advice or a story from one of my mentors or something I read in the past. The message will apply directly to my current situation, even though I wasn't able to relate or draw any parallels at the time.

Some questions to ask yourself: Which experiences or projects allowed you to make the largest impact? Which strengths or skills were you deploying to achieve those results? Do you have a coach or mentor that encourages you to step outside of your comfort zone? How often do you engage with leaders outside of healthcare who may inspire you to add value differently based on how they leverage their talents or strengths in other industries?

Allison

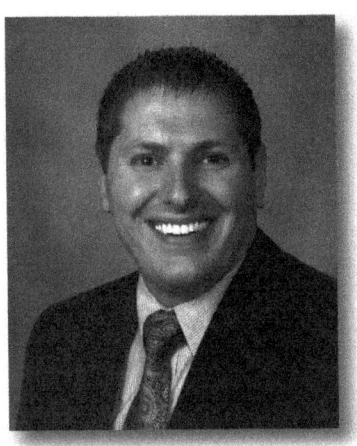

P. Zach White
PharmD

Finding Your Passion and Pursuing It with Vigor

Zach thought he was destined for retail pharmacy practice until he encountered his first PharmD advanced pharmacy practice experience (APPE) rotation in the neonatal intensive care unit (NICU). This experience transformed his life and career goals, leading him to find his career passion for pediatrics and neonatology. His pediatric expertise comes into play at home as he and his wife Amber raise two young children, Daxton (age 4) and Connor (age 1).

Zach is a clinical pharmacist in the NICU at Intermountain Healthcare's Utah Valley Hospital. He is the Women and Children's Pharmacy Team Lead, assisting in managing five pharmacists and one technician. He sits on three pediatric interdisciplinary committees, which make decisions for 22 Intermountain hospitals and 180 clinics. Zach received his PharmD from the University of Utah and completed a postgraduate year 1 (PGY1) residency at Mayo Eugenio Litta Children's Hospital in Rochester, Minnesota.

Zach's advice is: *Follow your passion and build on professional relationships. Passion provides the direction, and your professional relationships will lift you to where you want to be.*

Dear Pharmacy Colleague,

If you would have told me three-and-a-half years ago that I would be an inpatient pharmacist in a NICU, I would have replied that you are as crazy as Britney Spears was in 2007. My limited pharmacy experience and career path were founded completely in retail pharmacy. I had a strong interest in pediatrics, but a stronger interest in *not* doing a residency.

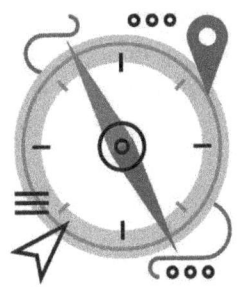

A railroad switch is a mechanical installation on the railroad track that allows a train to switch its course from the current track onto a new track. Stories have been shared about trains that were unintentionally left on a track, or inadvertently switched to a new track, arriving at train stations hundreds of miles from the intended destination. I feel that a railroad switch is the most appropriate analogy for my professional career plans between my last year of pharmacy school and today. Over the course of two years, I hit three major "switches" that changed my career course. These switches landed me in a metaphorical Chicago, instead of Atlanta.

THE FIRST SWITCH: RETAIL OR INPATIENT

In selecting your student and resident rotations, consider expanding beyond your comfort zone. The world of pharmacy is vast, and you might be pleasantly surprised when a new passion ignites.

I worked as a paid intern at a popular retail pharmacy chain during my last two-and-a-half years of pharmacy school. In selecting my APPE rotations, my approach was to choose as many pharmacy experiences as possible outside of retail pharmacy, as I figured I would have my entire career to become proficient in retail.

My first APPE opportunity was offered in the University of Utah Hospital NICU. I actually googled what NICU meant; because pediatrics was a strong interest, I jumped at the opportunity. Although my education was clinically focused, I did not have any clinical experience. For the entirety of the six-week rotation, I was overwhelmed and felt that I was always three feet underwater.

Despite the feeling of drowning, I found myself excited to come in each day to help the tiniest of patients. My incredible preceptor recognized my effort and, despite my rookie status, diligently spent much time mentoring me in all ways clinical. Additionally, we discussed his path through pharmacy school and residency and developed a similar plan for myself. Because I communicated my newfound passion for neonatology and put considerable effort into the rotation, my former preceptor contacted me to apply for a NICU clinical pharmacist position when it became available. My advice for you is to *consider each day on rotation like a job interview.* You never know when one of your preceptors will think of you for a job opportunity.

It took less than a week to realize that being a NICU pharmacist would be much more enjoyable for me than a job in retail pharmacy. I appreciated the dosing challenges and the variant pharmacokinetic profiles. There were disease states that I had never learned about, and the clinical decisions are often based on clinical judgment, as the literature in this population is often lacking. It took only two days on the rotation for my wife to notice how happy I was. "I can't believe how much happier you are—you must love it!" I replied that this would probably mean we would need to pursue residency training. Pursuing residency would drastically cut into our family time, which was extremely important to us. Her reply was: "If it is one or two extra years for you to be this happy, then it will be worth it in the long run, right?"

She was right.

THE SECOND SWITCH: RESIDENCY VERSUS NO RESIDENCY

When you find your passion, stop at nothing to make it a reality.

During my second pediatric APPE, I was waist-deep in residency application mud. My approach was to apply only for PGY1 programs at pediatric institutions. One APPE preceptor strongly discouraged this approach, as it would make the process more competitive. He counseled me to complete a PGY1 at any institution, and then apply for a PGY2 in pediatrics the following year to improve my chances at matching. However, I loved pediatric pharmacology so much that I wanted to get started helping in that patient population right away.

The application process was a whirlwind. ASHP Midyear was an incredible opportunity to trim down my application list from my initial list of 25 pediatric hospitals. I met with program directors and residents who provided clarity and gave me insight regarding their programs. I spent Christmas break writing letters of intent and finalizing the applications for the programs I wanted to apply to. As I interviewed at several places across the country, I focused on how I felt I would "fit" into their program. Match Day came, and I was blessed with the opportunity to pursue residency training at Mayo Eugenio Litta Children's Hospital in Rochester, Minnesota.

Residency is a deep-tissue massage—it hurts so good.

Residency wasn't easy—each night my wife and I would pray together and thank God that we were granted the mental and physical strength to be one day closer to completion. I viewed residency as a threat to my family time, and I felt like my three-year-old wouldn't recognize me by the end of the year. Because family time is so important to me, I made it a priority to be available for family dinner and spend time with them in the early evening before tackling residency projects and assignments in the twilight hours. Family time was more important than sleep.

But residency felt so right; I loved being immersed in pediatric pharmacology, and I loved my residency program. Mentors became friends, and residency provided opportunities that would not have been presented any other way. I was doing exactly what I wanted to do for a career.

THE THIRD SWITCH: PGY2 OR JOB

The major purpose of residency is to prepare you for your ideal job opportunity, whenever it presents. Notice all of your opportunities—both residency and job—at any given time.

While a PGY1 resident, I had the choice to pursue a PGY2 pediatric residency or to enter the job field. There were advantages to both choices. I felt that my PGY1 residency program would make me a competitive candidate for a PGY2. At the same time, I was ready to start providing for my young family and start my career.

My intention throughout my APPE rotations and into residency was to get hired onto the team at the University of Utah NICU, where my passion for neonatology was ignited. They did not require a PGY2 pediatrics residency. Frankly, if I could be competitive without one, I was ready to dive right in. It didn't take me long to realize that pursuing a job in my field of interest was more important to me than additional education.

For me, opportunity trumped education.

In November of my residency year, a friend and colleague from pharmacy school, who was doing his PGY1 at Utah Valley Hospital, texted me: "It's too bad you're in Minnesota; our NICU pharmacist of 18 years is retiring, and they are looking for a replacement." Because a clinical NICU pharmacist position opening is rare, I made my application a priority and fired up my résumé and a letter of intent. Even though I was still 8 months from finishing residency, I figured the more fishing lines that I had in the water, the more likely I would land a better catch.

My friend told me a few weeks later that the Utah Valley Hospital clinical manager took my application materials and asked him and one other resident, who I also went to pharmacy school with, whether or not I was a candidate worth pursuing. I remember sitting in my living room in Minnesota thinking: *What if I had slacked off on that pharmacy school project? Did I treat them with respect?* You never know when these professional relationships will come back to help or hurt you. Fortunately, I received a positive recommendation, and I was offered an opportunity to interview. I am confident that if they had not given a positive recommendation, I would not have been interviewed.

In the end, I was blown away by Utah Valley Hospital, their NICU, pharmacy management, and the opportunities for growth. I accepted their position immediately when it was offered.

REFLECTING ON THE RESIDENCY TO JOB TRANSITION

From my current vantage point working my dream job, I am so grateful I completed my residency training. The clinical experience, involvement in committees, research and quality improvement projects, and extensive presentation opportunities gave me the confidence and experience to hit the ground running in all aspects of my job.

When I moved back to Utah, I hiked to the top of a mountain 11,000 feet above sea level. There was a large rock on the edge of the steep slope, and my childish instinct kicked in—I pushed it down the steep slope. I watched it pick up momentum and crash down the mountain, smashing everything in its path. Likewise, this is how I viewed the transition between residency and the new job—the rock was already flying down the mountain, and I wanted to ride that momentum. The reduction in working hours between residency and my new job made it easy to keep a positive attitude. I was motivated to take on leadership responsibilities, pursue precepting opportunities, and tackle quality improvement projects. The more I stuck my head out from the everyday crowd, the more opportunities were presented. I said *yes* to as many opportunities as possible and rapidly became networked with big names at Intermountain Healthcare. I teamed up with them in solving problems. As credibility came, positions on corporate teams were offered. This snowballed to more opportunities and more "relationship capital."

Success in the early years of your career will come as you combine passion while building on professional relationships. Stay positive, be a good human. The future is as bright as you want it to be.

All the best,

Zach

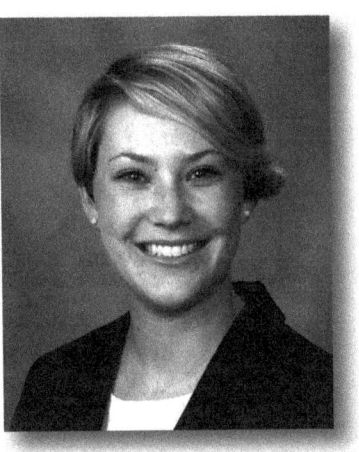

Kristyn Yemm
PharmD

Be Curious and Resilient

Kristyn is a bright, vivacious, energetic pharmacist with refreshing honesty about herself and her goals. She has in mind qualities of her ideal pharmacy practice, yet is open minded to clarification or revisions to her vision. Her curiosity is what makes her so interesting. Her curiosity keeps her asking questions: *Why do we treat this patient with this regimen, but not an analogous one? Why would you recommend this program to me and not another?* It is this curiosity which leads her to discover new ideas and solutions.

Kristyn is currently a Clinical Pharmacist on the Hematopoietic Stem Cell Transplant Service at the University of Washington Medical Center. She completed her accredited postgraduate year 2 (PGY2) oncology residency at the University of Washington Medicine in Seattle, Washington, and her accredited PGY1 pharmacy residency at the Mayo Clinic Hospital in Rochester, Minnesota. Kristyn received her BA in Biology at the University of North Carolina at Charlotte in Charlotte, North Carolina, and received her PharmD degree at the University of North Carolina, Eshelman School of Pharmacy in Chapel Hill, North Carolina.

Kristyn's advice is: **Listen to those who know you well and who have traveled the path before you. Embrace the challenges, lean into the obstacles, and you will find your way.**

Dear Pharmacy Colleague,

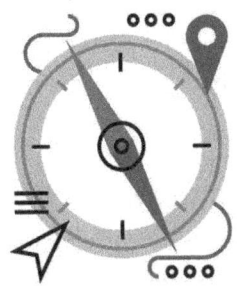

You are embarking on an exciting time in your career, although admittedly, it is one of the most intimidating times too. With the plethora of opportunities available in our profession, I remember how unsure I was about the path my career would take. I have always been a "slow, but steady" decision maker. I had identified long-term life goals, but choosing specific aspects of my future career was daunting. Interestingly, if you met me now, you might assume that my path was straightforward. I am currently in the specialty field of my greatest interest, but my journey has been one of resiliency. I owe much of my success to those who have mentored me over the years.

My advice to you at this point in your career is to keep an open mind, consult mentors, make a plan for your future, and be flexible to revise your plan. *Difficulties will arise, but with focused goals you will find yourself on a career path that you are passionate about.*

Be open to new opportunities and experiences. I entered my fourth year of pharmacy school with work experience only in retail pharmacy. I spent a few short weeks at a rural hospital in North Carolina and had never set foot into a large academic hospital. I knew that I enjoyed volunteering in the community, counseling patients at health fair events across the state, and working in a team setting, but I acknowledged that I had little insight into what was beyond this experience. I needed more exposure, so for my advanced pharmacy practice experiences I requested a wide variety of rotations in both the inpatient and outpatient settings. This resulted in assigned experiences in inpatient psychiatry, home infusion, cardiology intensive care, and oncology. However, one of my rotations was cancelled at the last minute, and I was assigned to two oncology rotations for back-to-back months. I felt this new challenge would amount to one of two things: give me time to build an oncology knowledge base or end up with a long 60-day experience waiting for my next rotation. These two months in oncology pharmacy ultimately spurred my interest for my future career. Not only did I realize I was passionate about oncology, but I also wanted to work in the inpatient setting.

Utilize mentors. Having mentors who will have deep conversations with you on a variety of topics is essential. As a student, I discovered my interest in oncology by September of my final year, and that second month on an oncology rotation solidified it. I will never forget sitting in my preceptor's office on a dreary Seattle afternoon in mid-October, toward the end of my rotation, telling him: "I just don't know if residency is for me." He had a knack for stating his opinions clearly and succinctly, and this conversation was no exception. "That's fine you think that Kristyn, but I am positive if you don't do a residency, you will get bored," he stated. It finally hit me. It made me stop and think: *What were my long-term goals?* To create a career practicing in a specialty setting, it would be necessary to do a residency. That conversation set the wheels in motion, and I started prepping for the ASHP Midyear Clinical Meeting (MCM).

Plan ahead. It is well known that the residency process gets more and more competitive. The number of outstanding candidates is growing coast to coast. Therefore, I did my due diligence. I selected ten programs with core values that aligned with my own to help me attain my career goals. I chose a range of programs that I felt qualified for, and one "dream big" program. I edited and re-edited my application and gave my letter-of-recommendation writers plenty of time. I left nothing to the last minute. I thought I had done all the right things to ensure everything would be ready on time.

Be prepared to change your plan. January first rolled around, and the flood of interview invitations began to hit the email boxes of students all around the country. Invitations slowly trickled in at first, but then picked up quickly as timed passed. I watched my fellow students talk excitedly about their upcoming interviews. I, too, had gotten one interview early on, and I quickly scheduled my accommodations. As time passed, I received that first rejection letter, then the second, and then by accident, one program sent me two rejection letters one week apart! Ten rejection letters later, I was in shock. I spent an evening filled with emotions stirring and swirling through me. My lone interview was my "dream big" program. I was dumbfounded. How could they have wanted to interview me but no one else had offered me an interview? I only had one shot. Was one shot enough? The field of candidates was so competitive. As I sat and contemplated, I devised a plan of attack for the future months. I had one interview. That was all I needed. I was going to go into this interview being completely myself. I researched the program and practiced my interview questions. I decided that I was interviewing this program as much as they were interviewing me. If it turned out that this program wasn't a good fit, I would enter the second residency match; if the second match didn't work out, I would apply for a job and re-apply the next year. Prepping my rank list was the easiest decision of my life. I was incredibly enthusiastic about the program I had interviewed with. My rank list was short, simple, and I was 100% confident that if I matched there it was a place I wanted to be. Match Day rolled around and, low-and-behold, I matched! I was one step closer to my career goals.

Accept that disappointments will come and go, but your goals can stay the same. As a first-year resident, I entered residency ready to pursue a PGY2 in oncology. I arranged my schedule to have an oncology rotation early in the residency year and prepared to apply to the early-commit program. My interview was scheduled just before the Thanksgiving holiday. I completely bombed the interview. I will never forget the feeling of stumbling through all of the questions and sweating through the presentation. I remember feeling like I was watching someone else interview for that position that day, because the person who interviewed wasn't me. After the interview, I knew I wouldn't get the position. My colleague, and good friend, got the position; he deserved it. I had broken my own interview mantra because I wasn't prepared.

After the holiday, I was notified that I hadn't been offered the position. I contacted my mentor, and we walked the mile loop of underground pathways in the hospital. We discussed the benefits of experiencing two different health systems, as she had during her training. My eyes were opened to the importance of being exposed to practice styles of different pharmacists. Armed with this insight, I applied nationally for a

PGY2 oncology specialty residency and interviewed with numerous programs. Match Day again rolled around, and again I was successful in matching with a program that would enable me to become an exceptional oncology pharmacist. I was encouraged by the positive outcome of the entire process. Having not been accepted into the early-commit program, I was able to network with oncology pharmacists across the country. That December, I participated in both MCM/Personnel Placement Service interviews and on-site interviews in the following months, which allowed me to explore what other institutions had to offer in the oncology specialty. I utilized this network again when I was pursuing jobs the following year.

My mentors had been right that residency was the path for me. Both my PGY1 and PGY2 residency programs have pushed my pharmaceutical knowledge beyond a level I could never have imagined. With residency training, I achieved skillsets beyond what could be self-taught. I attained skills in research, poster presentations, public speaking on a state and national level, teaching, and critical thinking. Today, as a practicing clinical pharmacist and new preceptor, I feel that my style is a sum of all of the places I have been and of all the preceptors who have taught me; but at the same time, it is quite uniquely me.

Examine your values and the roles in pharmacy that motivate you, and know that there are many different ways and opportunities to satisfy your passions within our field. Without the combined experience of PGY1 and PGY2 training, it would have been impossible to have the knowledge base and pharmacy tool box to be successful in my current position. My daily tasks include patient interactions with extensive medication counseling that I enjoyed so much from my early pharmacy career, combined with high-intensity work with an interdisciplinary team in an acute care setting in oncology.

Listen to those who know you well and who have traveled the path before you. Embrace the challenges, lean into the obstacles, and you will find your way.

Warm regards,

Kristyn